Lightening the
Shadow
DIAGNOSING AND LIVING WITH AN INVISIBLE CHRONIC ILLNESS

Darla Nagel

Cover design by Michael Brady Design

Copyright © 2018 Darla Nagel
All rights reserved. No part of this publication may be reproduced, stored in a retrieval system, or transmitted, in any form or by any means – electronic, mechanical, photocopy, recording, or otherwise – without prior written permission.

"Instant Relief," an excerpt from Chapter Four, was first published in *Patient Voice* (2016) and *Breath & Shadow* (2018).

No part of this book is to be construed as medical advice.

ISBN (paper): 978-0-692-14949-2
ISBN (ebook): 978-0-692-14950-8
Printed by IngramSpark

For Dr. MaryAnn Crawford and Dr. Lori Rogers, who are not medical doctors but who welcomed me to a therapeutic place

CONTENTS

Introduction: I'm Not Just Tired	*vi*
Chapter One: The Shadow Descends	1
Chapter Two: Medicines Fail to Lighten the Shadow	25
Chapter Three: Supplements Fail to Lighten the Shadow	45
Chapter Four: Naming the Shadow	63
Chapter Five: The Shadow Grows Heavier	103
Chapter Six: Lightening the Shadow	141
Bibliography	149
Appendix A: Seven Lessons for Living with a Chronic Illness	152
Appendix B: Resources for People with ME/CFS or Fibromyalgia	153
About the Author	155

INTRODUCTION:
I'm Not Just Tired
ॐ

I don't feel *tired*; I feel stunned on the ground from body slamming a brick wall. I feel fifty years older. I feel unplugged in the dark.

That's how I felt while combing my hair in the YMCA locker room after one of my hour-long swims. What I actually thought was *Maybe this is more than a cold. I'm whipped, and my legs are sore, even though I didn't swim as hard today.* Usually, swimming made me feel calm and strong, without causing sweating, even after the two-hour practices I'd done on my high school swim team.

"How are you doing, Darla?" asked another lap swimmer, who had been my journalism teacher in high school.

"All right. Just trying to shake off a cold," I answered.

"Are you home for the summer, then?"

"Yeah. I plan to take a couple online classes through Lansing Community College, though."

I also planned to work at McDonald's, a job I'd had for two years. But I'd had this cold, which was mild except for utter exhaustion that made me not want to do anything involving physical or cognitive effort, for a week now. I'd come down with it the Friday before Mother's Day of 2009, the day after I came home from my first year at Central Michigan University (CMU). I'd had a successful semester, declaring my major in English, completing eighteen credits with the hope of graduating a semester early, and being elected secretary of a writing club and an honor society.

I tucked my comb into my swim bag and said goodbye to my former teacher, whom I haven't seen since. *If I'm not better by Monday, I'll go see the doctor.*

I didn't know I would see many doctors: four internists, two neurologists, two endocrinologists, two rheumatologists, one alternative medicine doctor, one osteopathic doctor/certified naturopath, one psychiatrist, one cardiologist, one gynecologist, and one sleep medicine specialist. I didn't know I'd travel to various cities in my state, Michigan, to see them. I didn't know I would try treatment after treatment, including extra vitamins and minerals, vitamin B_{12} injections, antidepressants, a stimulant, herbal remedies, extra water, bed rest, pretending I was fine, taking fewer credit hours, quitting that McDonald's job, yoga, a therapeutic white noise machine, diet changes, environment changes, counseling, light therapy, oxygen therapy, you name it.

I didn't learn my diagnosis until two years and five months had passed and my condition had worsened. Two years represented a tenth of my life. Falling ill at age nineteen was like having my wings chopped off just as I was taking flight. Maybe the timing would've been worse if they had been chopped when I was hundreds of feet in the air, a year into a career in a city far from my parents. But I would've liked to soar through the air. My heart goes out to pediatric patients who will never fly on their own.

Plenty has been written about adopting a healthy lifestyle but not as much about adopting a chronically ill lifestyle. I've lightened the weight of my incurable illness enough to live a life that's of value to society and me. By sharing my experiences and seven major lessons I have learned, I will shine a light for my fellow patients and people without diagnoses and enlighten healthy people, especially doctors, about my invisible chronic illness. I don't pretend to have suffered more than other patients, but the ones who have suffered the most are too sick to speak out about this confounding illness and about how little health care professionals know about it.

CHAPTER ONE:
The Shadow Descends

☙

As I sat in the waiting room of my family's doctor, I was deciding how to describe my fatigue but couldn't concentrate. I'll call my internist Dr. One. (I'll change the names of doctors I say negative things about, along with some details about what we said in our interactions and about their appearances. I do not intend to harm them, and I recognize my bias and fallible memory.)

Dr. One had been my doctor since before I was born. He was about my parents' age. We liked his sense of humor, and he knew us more as people than as specimens.

I ended up telling him that I felt much like when I'd had mono a few years earlier, the only serious illness I'd had in my life. Based on my physical exam, nothing was wrong. Height 5'6", weight 122 pounds, no tenderness, no fever, no swollen glands, paler than many redheads but not in an unhealthy way, and so on. I looked much like the other woman sitting in the room, Mom. Same short, baby-fine blonde hair that requires an act of God to curl—Mom, unlike me, cares enough to wield perms and curling irons religiously to impose a bend on her hair. Same attractive legs, and same blue eyes, although I wear glasses.

Dr. One suspected that I had mono, which can strike more than once, he informed me, or some mystery condition that would resolve itself within a few weeks. He ordered some blood tests. In the meantime, he said to take a rest period, about fifteen minutes every morning and every afternoon, and to reduce the hours I worked. The blood tests came back normal.

I've never been able to sleep during the day, so I spent most of the rest periods listening to gentle music or praying. I was surprised I had enough to say to talk to God for fifteen minutes straight. The rests benefitted me spiritually but not physically. I tried going further by staying in bed for a few hours a day for a couple of weeks. This just reminded me that I was ill, then frustrated me when I felt no better after rising—and rising was suddenly challenging. When I told myself to get up when sitting or lying down, my body wouldn't obey. I sometimes leaned forward and shifted my weight to my feet. But then, I felt unable to move and unable to concentrate on the next step in the process. Next, I leaned back into the couch because that was more comfortable than sitting up. Or my thoughts wandered off. Then, I repeated my command to get up, usually with some progress but not enough to put me on my feet. The whole routine could take ten minutes, and the routine for forcing myself to get out of bed could take half an hour. On days when I had to wake by a certain time, I put my alarm clock as far from my bed as possible. Unless I was in public and there was urgency associated with the movement, such as getting off a bus when it reached my stop, I had to fight to exert myself.

I started writing down my activities and feelings in my personal journal, trying to find some explanation for my sudden illness. Journaling had been my way of recording memories and expressing feelings since third grade. I remember things best when I write them down, and I didn't want to forget to tell Dr. One about any patterns I noticed. Some days were harder than others, so I reread my entries from those days, trying to find out what made them worse. I noted that if I drank more than one cup of coffee or drank an espresso drink to give myself a boost the way I had while at school, I felt shaky, not energized. When the caffeine wore off, I often felt worse than I had before the drink. About once every other week, I had a day on which I was more energetic than usual. The problem with that was I tended to do so much on a good day that the next day was what I called a bad day, a day on which I felt much worse.

While journaling, I realized that the soreness in my back and neck I sometimes felt after work probably wasn't a result of that because I'd never had pain after work before. I wasn't sure whether I was having abnormal pain or my exhaustion was amplifying what would otherwise have been mild tenderness, like when being hungry while having a headache intensifies discomfort. I also noted multiple occurrences of a cruelly ironic phenomenon: trouble sleeping. I was exhausted, but it took an hour or two to fall asleep. It was like after a whole day of fighting fatigue, my body didn't know when to retreat and regroup. Or, I'd wake up before five o'clock, unable to go back to sleep.

The same week I noticed my frequent achiness, I had the first of countless occasional stomachaches right after eating. It wasn't a severe pain, closer to an annoyance, like the other sore areas I'd experienced. The exhaustion still concerned me much more. A shadow has no weight, but I felt like an invisible shadow was crushing me. If I knew what it was, its darkness would become less frightening. Maybe I'd even find a way to make the shadow fade.

I'd heard of chronic fatigue syndrome (CFS) back when I had battled mono and a member of my extended family had joked that he thought only members of a certain race got it. *Chronic fatigue syndrome* was the only phrase I could think of to type into Google to investigate what could be ailing me. I did, and by skimming the first few websites I found, I saw there was a range of symptoms of and beliefs about this illness. Plus, it had other names: myalgic encephalomyelitis and chronic fatigue and immune dysfunction syndrome. Some sources considered it the same as fibromyalgia. I doubted they were the same. One of Mom's bosses (Mom works two part-time jobs) has fibromyalgia, and I wasn't in nearly enough pain for that to be my problem. I soon felt drained just reading about never-ending fatigue and closed the browser.

On another day of research, I read and printed an article about CFS on the Mayo Clinic's website. According to the article, CFS had no diagnostic test. It could be diagnosed only after every possible cause of my lack of energy had been eliminated. I had no idea how long that elimination process could take. CFS had lots of symptoms, many of which I didn't have, so I decided to research other medical conditions.

Thinking back to my high school biology class, I remembered that mitochondria make energy for cells. I wondered if some problem with them was causing my weariness. Another Internet search showed that mitochondrial diseases exist, but I lacked the key symptoms of muscle weakness and decreased mobility. That train of thought had hit a dead end. Instead, I considered everything that had happened in the month before I became ill, desperate to find some unusual triggering stress or event, even though I didn't worry or stress a lot about life's troubles. I asked Mom for her ideas as she washed dishes and I dried and put them away. We often have good conversations while doing this chore.

"We found out Grampa had colon cancer that month," she pointed out. "But that's been worrying me more than it's worried you."

"Mm-hmm. God's going to do whatever is best for Grampa, and Gramma." I thought some more. "I donated blood during the last week of the semester, but I called the

Red Cross yesterday. They said if I didn't have any symptoms within twenty-four hours after donating, that's not causing my problems." I slid steak knives into the knife block.

"Doing eighteen credits and two jobs wasn't that much of a strain, right?"

"No. I wasn't working full-time. Only two of my exams were remotely hard. My senior year was much worse, with everything I was doing: running the newspaper without a staff adviser, the musical, president of SADD, two after school choirs . . ."

"Yeah, that was nuts. I don't know how you did that." Mom dunked a pan. "You don't think your roommates did something, do you? Slipped something into your water, or . . . I don't know."

My roommates had acted as though I didn't exist, but I told Mom, "No. They weren't nice, but they weren't *that* mean. And why would I have symptoms now that I'm away from them? It didn't start until the day after I got home."

Mom rinsed the pan and said, "I sure hope you have better roommates this year. I don't want to see you go back to that. I don't know how we're going to pay for it, anyway. That $8,000 scholarship you had last year really helped."

She'd been worrying about college costs since April, so I reminded her, "I still have my Board of Trustees Scholarship for $2,000, and I should hear soon if I got any of the others I applied for. We have another month until the first bill for next year is due."

"Right. I shouldn't be worrying. Maybe all my worrying is causing your problems. You're stressing out being here at home with me."

"No, Mom. It's not you. You've never been demanding or made me stress out. I'm the one who's hard on myself. You're helping me, and you believe something's wrong with me. Unlike Dad." He seemed to think my illness was something simple that would pass soon.

When I mentioned my new symptoms and the lack of an emotional trigger during the follow-up appointment, Dr. One presented another idea: that my exhaustion was related to my polycystic ovary syndrome, which he'd diagnosed over a year ago. That sounds scary, right? All it means in my case is that I have irregular periods. He ordered a pelvic ultrasound, which showed no problems, and started me on birth control pills to regulate my cycle. The idea was that making my hormones fluctuate normally would undo any hormonal cause of the exhaustion. But one cycle later, instead of feeling better, I'd recorded two new symptoms.

The first was general cognitive difficulty. I dreaded going to my job at McDonald's now because handling stress, concentrating, thinking fast, and remembering things were problematic. I'd once prided myself on my ability to minimize worries and stress. But one evening as I ran the busy drive-thru, the coworker handing orders out the window told me I'd forgotten to put napkins in the bag I'd just handed her. All I had to do was grab a few napkins from the holder in front of me, take a step to the table where I'd set the bag, and put them in. Instead, I snatched an empty bag, chucked a few napkins into it, and practically threw it at her, saying something like "Well, put . . ." without being able to think of what I wanted to say. Then I yanked my headset off, told a less busy coworker to cover for me for a few minutes, and darted to the bathroom, thinking I was going to scream or cry. But too worn out to do either, I gripped the edges of the counter to support myself rather than sit on the floor. I stared at the sink until a manager came in to see what was wrong, and I couldn't think of anything stronger to tell her than "I'm so tired." On other shifts, my memory was a bigger problem than handling stress. I knew darn well how many squirts of syrup went in an iced mocha, but my mind sometimes went blank after I'd scooped ice into the cup. Worse yet, sometimes I was momentarily unsure why I held a cup of ice as another order blared through my headset, as a chorus of beeps pierced my ears, as a distant manager shouted something to the person next to me.

These cognitive challenges continued outside work. When I took an exam for the one online class through the community college that I hadn't dropped, I found myself reading many questions three times before they sank in. This was frightening because reading holds special power and pleasure for me. I first distinguished myself from my peers during kindergarten by reading to the class when my teacher lost her voice. I've always learned best by reading and remembered a high percentage of what I read. At home, my brain continued upsetting me. I entered rooms with no recollection of what I'd meant to do there. I went into the kitchen to get a snack and returned to my bedroom with a bottle of water instead more than once. Now, for a middle-aged person with too much on his or her mind or for someone with ADHD, this memory and concentration difficulty is probably normal, but I was only nineteen. Sometimes, I had trouble putting two pieces of information together to generate a third piece. I remember sitting down for dinner once, seeing a fork and a plate of food, and knowing I was supposed to do something with the fork and food but not immediately knowing what. I wondered whether this was what it was like to have a traumatic brain injury, but I hadn't hit my head recently.

The second new symptom was just plain bizarre. Shortly before I fell asleep one night, my left foot twitched. I rolled over, hoped it wouldn't twitch again or cramp, and fell asleep. From then on, any time I was relaxed, I tended to twitch. Sometimes, it happened to one finger, and other times, it happened to a muscle group, like my thigh. When I allowed Dr. One to watch this sensation while I relaxed in the examination room during the next appointment, he referred me to a neurologist.

The problem with being referred to a specialist was the wait. By now, August had come, which brought on worrying. I didn't want to go back to school because I wasn't sure that I could handle the sixteen credits I'd signed up for. I had already quit my job as a staff reporter for the college newspaper and decided to work at McDonald's every other weekend so that I wouldn't have to make the ninety-minute drive home to Flushing as often. Driving was particularly draining. I also considered quitting a new campus job I'd secured at the end of the previous school year: writing consultant at the Writing Center. A writing center is a place for students to get feedback that makes them stronger writers. Quitting that job sounded like a more reasonable way to make life easier than dropping a class.

I shared this idea with Mom during a walk down our street in Flushing, a quiet suburb of Flint with about 8,000 residents. We agree on almost anything, from food choices—chocolate and more chocolate—to clothing choices—no shoes with heels higher than an inch. But this time, she disagreed with my idea.

"No! It'll be such good experience," she reminded me.

I knew working to make students better writers would be valuable. After all, I planned to have a career at a publishing company in Chicago or another Midwestern metropolitan area. I wanted to be within driving distance of my parents, and New York City sounded too big and crowded to me. I figured I'd start as an editorial assistant and work my way into copyeditor and project editor positions until I reached the managing editorial level.

"How about working the smallest possible number of hours per week?" Mom suggested. "How many is that?"

"Six. Even so, I'm not sure that'll be enough to make this semester doable."

"Well, don't work so hard in the classes that aren't for your major," Mom advised.

I usually took her advice, even though she sometimes added this disclaimer after giving my brother or me advice pertaining to college: "I don't know. I never went to college." Dwight, who is three years older than I am, was in college in Kentucky, having moved there and spent a couple of years working after high school. Mom had never needed to push me to do well in school. We're both hardworking. She worked two part-time jobs and, with my help, still provided homemade dinners six or seven nights a week. I'd been helping her around the house since my first attempt to unload the dishwasher at age two. Several times, she had told me we were so alike that she felt sorry for me.

"Guess I'll keep praying my classes are easy this semester," I said. "I know Dad wouldn't like it if I quit the job." I was thinking about the dose of silent treatment he had given me earlier that summer.

He'd gotten mad because my car, a beloved light blue '89 Cadillac (picture a slightly boxy boat), was spotted with dirt and bug poop from parking it under a box elder tree in the front yard. He'd assumed that I hadn't washed my car because I didn't care about it. The truth was that I'd been waiting for a day when I had enough energy left after work to go to the car wash, which was an uncomfortable task. I was always dripping sweat after work, and the car's air-conditioning didn't work. Dad, a GM mechanic and genius when it comes to cars, had promised to try fixing it.

"Why should I bother working on that AC when you don't even try to keep the car clean?" Dad had asked one afternoon.

"I've been so tired! I really want to wash it," I had answered, my voice growing higher pitched. "Look, I'll do it first thing tomorrow morning, before work, when it's cooler." My shift would start at six o'clock in the morning. That obvious solution had only just popped into my head, showing that I hadn't been thinking clearly lately.

His response had been a shake of his head, a (justified) grumble about how I should've done it about a week ago, and the silent treatment for the rest of that day and the next. Mom's response had been writing down three verses from the Bible that she had happened to read and putting them on the kitchen counter with my coffee the next morning: "He gives strength to the weary and increases the power of the weak. Even youths grow tired and weary, and young men stumble and fall; but those who hope in the LORD will renew their strength. They will soar on wings like eagles; they will run and not grow weary, they will walk and not be faint" (Isaiah 40:29–31). These verses have become my favorite portion of the Bible because of the comfort they offer a "tired and weary" youth like me, and Mom's index card with these verses remains on the center of my bulletin board at home.

During our walk, Mom reassured me, much like she had then: "Your dad will accept this eventually. He knows you're sick but doesn't realize just how sick." She held my hand for the next few steps. "Try not to worry about him. The stress will only make things worse."

It had to be hard for my parents to accept such a drastic change in me, but Dad's dull perception of the effects of my illness frustrated me. True, Mom and I tend to have the same thought at the same time. Before friends and roommates met her, I told them she was like me, just taller and better. She nearly always understands my perspective because of our nearly identical personalities and because we share a zeal for Jesus that Dwight and Dad reserve for Christmas and Easter. I'm more comfortable talking about my body with Mom than with Dad because she's a woman. I'm quiet and introverted, whereas Dad is talkative and outgoing. Nearly anywhere we go—once even in Silverton, Colorado—he finds someone he knows. But I always told him what happened during doctor's appointments, and I wasn't acting stronger than I felt when he was around.

I can understand why he reacted this way. Ever since I became ill, I've looked better than I've felt. This has been a blessing and a curse. It's been nice not having people gawk at me or fear touching or talking to me. But people, including doctors, have underestimated how ill I am because as a quiet, smiley person, I can hide my suffering without trying to. Sometimes I'm quiet because I lack the energy to converse. My glasses even hide the dark circles I often have under my eyes.

During the weeks before my neurologist appointment, I researched some more. I tried typing in all my symptoms to see what Google would find, having read in *Good Housekeeping*, Mom's favorite magazine, about a woman who did so and figured out what was wrong with her. The first result was from www.rightdiagnosis.com. This website allowed me to select symptoms from a list and see what illnesses caused all of them. I knew just about any illness had fatigue as a symptom, so I selected insomnia, difficulty concentrating, muscle pain, and digestive trouble instead. I wasn't surprised to see depression, CFS, and fibromyalgia listed in the dozens of matches. Most of the other matches were cancers or thyroid problems. I didn't know what Addison's disease and adrenal insufficiency were, however. After another Google search showed me they concerned the endocrine system, the glands and hormones that regulate the body, I decided that seeing an endocrinologist wouldn't hurt.

After waiting over a month to see the neurologist and a few weeks to see an endocrinologist, I had no answers. Both specialists basically said, "I don't know. You seem fine to me. On the plus side, there's nothing seriously wrong with you." *Nothing seriously wrong!*

When the nurse took my blood pressure at the endocrinologist's office, it was something like 90 over 50, much lower than my normal numbers. Mom and I thought it must've been a bad reading. Neither the nurse nor the endocrinologist mentioned it, however. More bothersome was when the endocrinologist suggested toward the end of the appointment that there could be a psychological cause of my illness. I absolutely did *not* have depression or another mental health disorder. Shortly after leaving the endocrinologist's office, what I should've responded with popped into my head: "Try being me for a week, and see how you like it! Then see if you still think nothing's seriously wrong!"

The specialists didn't understand the stress and, at times, torment I experienced from adjusting to college life in my condition and from forcing myself *not* to put my best effort into my classes. I called home two or three times in tears because I couldn't keep up with my work and class schedule. Mom drove me home for a weekend twice because I didn't feel up to driving, and she sent me back to school with a pan of homemade granola bars or other high-protein food for my breakfasts. I dropped my math class and took my German class on a credit/no credit basis. It dawned on me that my ailment wasn't easy to diagnose, because if it had been, a doctor would've figured it out by now. I was frequently cold, like my body didn't have enough energy to keep me warm. I enjoy singing, so I often hum. But sometimes, I noticed I was absently humming some unrecognizable, brief, repetitive tune.

With time, it became a signal that I needed to stop doing whatever was draining me.

My cognitive challenges were worsening. I wasn't as smart as I used to be. Homework took me about twice as long as it had the previous semester. I had been able to work on a paper for two hours in one sitting then, not that I recommend writing for that long without a break. Now, either my attention wandered to my dorm's gray-tiled floor, or the meaning of a sentence didn't sink in until the second or third time I read it. Some nights when I wrote in my journal before going to sleep, I couldn't focus enough to write complete sentences. Writing in complete sentences didn't matter in my journal the way it did in papers for English classes, but I still didn't like my brain's apparent decline.

My vision of my future became less and less clear, like looking at a landscape as the sun is setting. The heavy shadow engulfed my plans to ace my classes and secure an editorial internship in Chicago for the following summer. I now fully understood the saying "If you have your health, you have everything" (but reminded myself that it would be more accurate to replace *health* with *faith*). Without good health, each day was a battle, and the future didn't look any better. I was now a worrier. Every time something unusual happened with my body, I worried. *My hands are shaking. Is this a new symptom? I have a headache again. Is this normal?* More often than I'd like to admit, I worried that I was going to collapse, maybe die, because of something the doctors were missing.

Adjusting to being chronically ill was like repeating my early teen years: my family and friends weren't always sure how to react to me, my body was doing weird things, and I had no idea what my future held.

On top of that, a new symptom developed in October: excessive sweating. One night, I woke up soaked. I hadn't had a nightmare, and my pajamas weren't too heavy for that time of year. The next day, I perspired at work. Neither I nor the Writing Center was warm. After all, the Writing Center location I was in that day was in a basement. I wasn't nervous or anything; instead, I was having fun. Both the night sweats and excessive sweating became nearly daily occurrences. I quickly learned to use clinical-strength deodorant and carry another shirt to change into in my backpack. With the insomnia, night sweats, and homework, I rarely got a good night's sleep, which was what I needed most.

I had another appointment with Dr. One on a Friday in November. I asked whether there were other tests I should have.

"I've ordered every relevant blood test," he replied. "Maybe we should think about this in a different way." He talked about how people have various moods that can affect them in various ways. "I'd like to refer you to a psychiatrist. It's possible you have some kind of mood disorder."

"A mood disorder?" I asked. "This isn't all in my head."

"She can't drive," Mom piped up, and Dr. One spun on his stool to face her.

"She can't drive?" he echoed, sounding incredulous.

"I had to drive up and get her from CMU this morning," Mom said sternly. "And when I got there, she looked about too tired to stand up." Mom had even lugged my suitcase, heavy with dirty laundry, to the car and had lifted it into the trunk for me.

"Look, I'm not saying this is all in your head, Darla," Dr. One insisted, turning back to face me. "Since I can't make a diagnosis, I'd like to rule out psychological causes and prescribe a mood medicine for you."

He made it sound like this was the only option, so I gave in and told him to make the referral and write the prescription. Then, I started to cry out of frustration. Mom came over and hugged me with tears in her eyes. His demeanor didn't change.

I was sick of seeing doctor after doctor without getting answers or empathy. I yearned for a name for the shadow and imagined taping the name to a dartboard and attacking it with darts. I searched my memories, asking whether some event had harmed me psychologically. Had I pushed myself too hard to get As in school for all these years? Was I too close to Mom? Was I experiencing delayed effects of my brother's ceaseless teasing or Dad's alcoholism when I was younger? He'd been sober for five years, ever since he'd developed a still undiagnosed condition that causes him to vomit until there's only bile left to throw up whenever he consumes alcohol or certain processed foods.

Meanwhile, winter's chill entered me and froze anything resembling hope. More likely what was happening was the antidepressant—what Dr. One had called a mood medicine—was having the opposite effect. I didn't have proof until years later. I kept pulling at my hair and stroking my chin, two nervous habits I'd never had before. I counted my blessings, but that just made me feel guilty for feeling down. I cried and felt worthless daily. My life seemed pointless. After all, I was at school to learn. If I wasn't learning much, what was I doing there, and if I didn't get my degree, what kind of future could I have? I didn't want to eat. All I wanted to do was sleep. The fear that I'd collapse and die because of something the doctors had missed became a wish. Please, if you ever sink into the pool of symptoms in this paragraph, get help. I didn't right away.

During a writing club meeting, when responding to the creative writing prompt, "Write anything about joy," I struggled to write, even when I resorted to freewriting, which is writing whatever comes to mind without stopping. I wrote, "All I think about is my sadness. My pen feels limp in my hand. It is lifeless, after all. Freewriting fails me today. I'm killing a tree for worthless human folly." *Failure* was a word I thought often. I'd failed to figure out what was wrong and to live the way I had when I'd been healthy. Before then, I'd been blessed to have been spared from failure, except for algebra tests and quizzes in eighth grade, but those hadn't affected my family and identity the way this illness had. I didn't want to live like this anymore. I wasn't my smiley, ambitious self anymore. The person I was now wanted to sleep and never wake.

That person terrified me during a rest period one afternoon. She was alone in her dorm, sitting at her desk in front of the window currently covered by the curtain, spending her habitual fifteen minutes of afternoon rest praying. She prayed, "God, please kill me." She opened her eyes in surprise, and her heart conveyed its will to live by pumping faster. *I deserve to die just for praying that.* But moments passed without her dying. *Well, you're sparing me, God. Please forgive me. If I have that desire again, I'll call the campus counseling center.*

But that person still made it clear to the psychiatrist, when they met two days later, that this depression was a result, absolutely not the cause, of my undiagnosed illness. The psychiatrist wrote to Dr. One to explain this truth and ask him to reevaluate me and prescribe a different antidepressant.

The second day I took the new medicine, the Saturday after Thanksgiving, I was on my knees to get something from under my bed when Mom called for me from the kitchen. *What the heck does she need now? I'm busy here!* I thought, settling for grumbling incoherently rather than yelling at her. As I got to my feet, my brain slid to my left, so I grabbed the edge of my desk. But I wasn't falling. Also, it struck me that this was the second time today that I'd felt like yelling over something minor, when I couldn't remember the last time I'd been mad enough to yell. *This isn't me. What's going on?* A headache followed. When the sliding sensation happened again the next couple of times I changed the position of my head, I called the psychiatrist, afraid to continue taking the medicine. She had me wean off it.

My family spent December waiting for Dr. One's office to contact us. And waiting. The next antidepressant I tried wasn't much better. I had the worst Christmas I've ever had. I remember hearing the song "All Is Well" at a concert and crying, apparently upset with myself for being unhappy. Christmas was the first time I'd seen Dwight since becoming ill, and he must have noticed how little energy I had to help Mom. Instead of ignoring his teasing or using sarcasm to deflect it like I usually did, I snapped at him. I had time for my hobbies but didn't enjoy them. I lacked the energy to swim much and the concentration to sing, write, or scrapbook for long.

Once January arrived, Dad became angry about the lack of follow-up from Dr. One. Most people who know Dad avoid ticking him off because his temper makes his behavior unpredictable. He knew a psychiatrist wasn't what I needed, and he could see something was physically wrong. In fact, I'd decided to take a leave from McDonald's next semester because the combination of the drive home and the work was unbearable. Dad made an appointment to, as he put it, "make that jerk aware that he isn't helping you any."

A few days into the new semester, I was heading out of my residence hall complex for an afternoon class when my phone rang. It was Dad. He was angry, but that tone was common when he called from work because GM's management was enough to make anyone miserable. Dad said he'd met with Dr. One yesterday after work to discuss why we hadn't heard from him. I set my backpack on the floor and pulled off my Mom-knitted hat, figuring this would last longer than our usual three-minute-long phone calls.

"The first thing he said was 'Your daughter is completely gaga,'" Dad articulated, sounding like he was trying to restrain rage.

"Oh," I answered flatly, hoping Dad would say something to help me understand.

"I didn't say anything," Dad continued. "I just showed him that thing you had in the newspaper, the one about the scholarship."

I'd received another scholarship at the beginning of the semester, and the *Flint Journal* had written a brief about it.

"The doc said, 'That's great. Good for her.' I wanted to punch him. But I didn't, I just sat there. He didn't say a word."

Then, Dad told Dr. One that there was no point in my seeing him again.

Dr. One's answer was "Probably not. Your bitchy wife barely lets her talk when she's here."

"*What?*" I exclaimed. I wasn't all that upset at being called gaga. I'd already reasoned, on some night when I hadn't been able to sleep, that Dr. One didn't care about me. But insulting Mom, the best mom and my best friend, was infuriating. I talked more than Mom during my appointments—she jumped in only when my mind went blank. I switched my attention back to Dad, who was still talking.

"I was out of that chair, my hand in a fist. 'You will not refer to my wife in that manner,' I said. But I knew I'd be in trouble if I hit him, so I told him, 'You're not going to see any of us again,' and got the hell out of there."

I could picture Dad in his Carhartt coat and plaid flannel shirt, raising a fist smeared with grease. Maybe his blue eyes had turned gray, that creepy sign that he is enraged. I sat on the floor, and Dad retold the story, filling in some details, like the way Dr. One's eyes had widened in surprise when Dad had stood up. I was proud of Dad for confronting Dr. One without beating him up. As I told Dad shortly before I had to hang up and rush to class, that jerk wasn't worth being arrested over.

Although I was far more upset about his insult of Mom, I still felt violated by Dr. One. I'd trusted him to look at and in me and to help me. I thought doctors were supposed to care about people and be curious enough to investigate causes of symptoms. I didn't see how I could trust another one. But on the bright side, this situation made it clear that my illness wasn't the result of anything in my mind. The depression lightened up within weeks due to this new understanding and the continuation of a few other activities I'd started that year. The first was seeing a counselor on campus to talk through my feelings, and the second was befriending two of my roommates, twins who were a year older than I. The third was taking an antidepressant that didn't cause extreme headaches, irritability, or other side effects. Smiling felt less like having a slice of lemon between my lips and teeth.

CHAPTER TWO:
Medicines Fail to Lighten the Shadow
☙

Mom and Dad asked around, hoping someone knew a good doctor. I posted a plea for doctor recommendations on my Facebook page and was surprised when no one responded. Maybe there were no good doctors in the area. Flushing is a small suburb of Flint, which in several ways isn't a nice city to live in, so I couldn't blame doctors for not wanting to live around here. Dad found the next doctor. I'll call him Dr. Two.

According to one of the guys Dad carpooled with, Dr. Two, another doctor in a family medicine practice, was aggressive in finding out what was wrong with patients. Plus, Dr. Two took our new insurance. Dad had switched our family's health insurance plan after discovering a possible reason so few doctors accepted our old insurance plan: after a certain number of doctor visits by one household in one year, the company wouldn't pay the doctor. Maybe that explained why Dr. One had done less during our final appointments. I was grateful Dad took the initiative there.

During the monthlong wait for my appointment, the result of the new semester more than Dr. Two's schedule, my worries stewed. Maybe he wouldn't have any answers or treatments, either. I read the copy of my medical records from Dr. One that Dad had obtained, trying to find a lab result that was close to abnormal or something he'd overlooked. My white blood cell count was too low, I discovered. I knew a high white blood cell count meant infection, but I didn't know what a low one meant and couldn't find an answer that fit my other symptoms online. I also looked up medical terms from the blood test reports online, like *reticulocyte* and *basophil*, but the definitions didn't lead me to any guess as to a diagnosis.

The neurologist had called my jerking "low-amplitude myoclonic twitching" in his report, so I looked that one up online, too. It wasn't associated with any particular illness and usually resulted from stress, which didn't make sense because I twitched when I was relaxed. Another dead end in my research. Dr. One's note regarding my twitching stood out to me because of its use of underlining: "seems <u>voluntary</u>." Apparently, he'd decided even then that I was a basket case. I wondered why he'd bothered referring me to the neurologist and endocrinologist and whether he'd tainted their perception of my condition's severity.

This brings me to my first lesson learned to share with people with undiagnosed or chronic illnesses: *examine medical records to see if there's an abnormal result the doctor missed or something he or she is trying to hide.* Plus, the more I know about what's happening to my body, the better I understand what doctors say and what treatments they give.

Frustrated, curious, and still investigating what was wrong, I returned to the Mayo Clinic's chronic fatigue syndrome (CFS) article that I'd printed. The first time I'd read it, I'd thought I needed to have the entire list of symptoms to receive that diagnosis. Now I saw that I'd misunderstood the list, but I still wasn't sure whether I fit the diagnostic criteria: fatigue not caused by other mental or physical conditions or by life situations, not relieved by rest, causing substantial reduction in activities, and lasting six or more months (check!), as well as four of the following:

◊ worsened fatigue after mental or physical exertion (check!)
◊ new kind of headaches (nope)
◊ loss of memory or concentration (check!)
◊ sore throat (nope)
◊ tender, enlarged lymph nodes (nope)
◊ pain switching from one joint to another without swelling (nope)
◊ trouble sleeping (check!)
◊ unexplained muscle pain (maybe—it wasn't a daily occurrence, so did it count?)

I saw a close enough match to the criteria to continue reading about CFS. The outlook of this illness wasn't encouraging. Some patients improve with age, some worsen with age, and some experience a cycle of improvement and then worsening, improvement and then worsening. CFS usually strikes in middle age, and about four times more women than men are diagnosed with it. Severe cases confine patients to bed, but patients with mild cases may be able to work full-time with accommodations. Treatment options include stimulants, antidepressants, antivirals, and a sugar called D-Ribose.

A fact sheet from the Chronic Fatigue Immunodeficiency Syndrome Association of America, now called the Solve ME/CFS Initiative, gave more detail on the outlook. ME stands for myalgic encephalomyelitis, another name for CFS. About half of patients improve with treatment, and approximately 5 percent recover fully. CFS's cause is unconfirmed but seems to be a complicated mix of problems with brain chemicals, hormones, and the immune system. Everything I read made me hope I had a more easily curable illness.

In February 2010, I had my first appointment with Dr. Two. Most of the exam room's tan wall space had posters that weren't enough to read while waiting . . . and waiting . . . to see him: one poster for frequent urination, one for the effects of smoking, one for arthritis, and one for hypothyroidism. Mom and I kept rereading the last one because the symptoms sounded much like what I had, even though I'd had at least two blood tests to check for thyroid problems. No magazines. I wondered whether he did any leisure reading. I'm an avid reader, so not having reading material made me unsure about him.

Mom relaxed and smiled when he poked his head into the room, saying cheerfully, "Hi. Hold the phone. I'll be in soon."

Dr. Two came back not long afterward and talked with Mom and me for about ten minutes. He was short, had curly black hair, wore a silver class ring, and looked younger than Dr. One, in his forties instead of fifties. I tried to determine through his body language whether he was trustworthy. He had read my medical records, which pleased me because it had taken Dad time and effort to get them from Dr. One's office. I gave Dr. Two a typed timeline of my illness that listed when each symptom had begun, when I'd seen each specialist, and when I'd started and stopped each medication. The timeline benefitted me as much as it did him because I'd lost track of when each event had occurred. Lesson two for anyone with a chronic or undiagnosed illness is to *compile such a timeline.* I eventually learned to keep two timelines: a full one for my reference and a two-page version with only the most important events to give to doctors because their time is limited.

Dr. Two listened more than he took notes. Nothing was psychologically wrong, other than depression resulting from my illness, he declared. *Bingo*, I thought. He realized that I wasn't crazy after just ten minutes of talking with me. Dr. One's so-called diagnosis sounded even sillier now, considering he had known me my whole life. And that wasn't the only good news. Dr. Two had plenty of ideas for investigating what was wrong, and he told me some while flicking his pen back and forth rapidly between two fingers. He had enough ideas to where I didn't see any reason to ask about CFS.

He had my blood tested for Lyme disease and for heavy metals that I could've been exposed to at McDonald's or from the well water at home, but the test results were normal. Also, he referred me to a cardiologist. He assured us he heard nothing unusual when listening to my heart, but any problem with my lungs or heart would cause my debilitating exhaustion. Fortunately, the cardiologist's first words to me were "You're too young to be here." My electrocardiogram showed that my cardiovascular system was fine.

Another one of Dr. Two's ideas was to prescribe me a stimulant. It seemed to give a tiny energy boost, so I asked Dr. Two during my next appointment whether I could increase the dose. The only problem with taking the stimulant was the extra paperwork involved. I don't know whether this is true nationwide, but in Michigan, doctors cannot write prescriptions that include refills for this stimulant. Every month, doctors have to write a new scrip. Plus, our insurance company required Dr. Two to fill out a prior authorization form before I could get the medicine. When Dr. Two increased the dose, I found out the hard way that he needed to complete a new prior authorization form. However, the hassle became worthwhile when I regained about 10 percent of my functioning by taking the stimulant.

The next month, Dr. Two prescribed a prenatal multivitamin, saying this was the best kind of multivitamin a woman my age could take, and another medicine called Savella. He seemed to be in a hurry and wasn't clear about what the medicine was supposed to do. Its information sheet said it was for treating fibromyalgia. I couldn't see why Dr. Two would've prescribed it if he didn't think I had fibromyalgia or something similar. But I couldn't have that because my pain wasn't intense or a daily occurrence. Muscle or joint pain happened only when I overdid it physically.

Neither the multivitamin nor Savella helped, so the next month I told Dr. Two exactly that. I asked him whether he thought I had fibromyalgia.

"No. *Fibromyalgia* is not a term I use in my practice," he replied. "I can see that some of the symptoms seem to be real. There can be problems with the nervous system that cause a lot of pain or fatigue. Savella is supposed to address problems with nerves, so that's why I gave it to you. But if it's not helping, wean off it."

"Okay," I said, surprised that he didn't believe that fibromyalgia was real. Knowing that boss of Mom's who has it had shown me the disease was real a long time ago. I was curious about his position but more curious about what his next idea for me was. I asked, "So, what do we do now?"

He referred me to another neurologist and a gynecologist. I wish that I had asked for his reason for the referral to the neurologist. In retrospect, I suspect that he hadn't noticed the report from the first neurologist in my medical records. The second neurologist ordered an MRI of my brain to check for any abnormality there. I supposed a brain abnormality would throw my body out of whack.

Having the top third of my body inside a metal doughnut on its side, like some spaceship's escape pod, was eerie. My glasses were off, so the little window positioned above eye level didn't give me a clear view of my legs and the outside world. I tried to stay still when there was a sound like nails being hammered into random spots on the machine, then whirring as metal parts shifted, then more hammering, over and over, for about a half hour. I was definitely ready to get out when it was over. About a week later, the neurologist showed me the pictures of my perfectly normal brain, although my eyeballs seemed huge, protruding from a mess of white and gray blobs. My first thought was that I was disappointed that I still had no diagnosis. Further showing the brain's mysteriousness, my next thought was: *at last, I have evidence that I have a brain to show to my brother.*

With that appointment done, I waited for the one with the gynecologist, which I'd requested because I'd had a benign but daily vaginal discharge since the first week of my illness, maybe even the first day. Dr. One had done a pelvic exam and found nothing abnormal, but I wanted a specialist's opinion now that the discharge had continued for so long. However, the gynecologist also found nothing wrong.

During another visit to Dr. Two in May, I read a sign in the waiting room about a policy change that annoyed me because it meant that I couldn't take Mom in with me anymore: "Dr. Two sees his adult patients alone. If you have a condition that makes it impossible for you to enter the exam room by yourself, please notify the receptionist." The policy didn't affect me during that appointment because Mom had had to work, but it made my stomach feel funny and certainly didn't seem ethical.

I always liked having Mom with me. For one thing, she was usually my driver. Dad commuted nearly an hour to work every day, so it worked better for Mom to take me to appointments. Both of her bosses were kindhearted people who were reasonable about letting her take an hour or two off, especially once Mom told them I was having health problems. Also, driving exhausted me to the point where I didn't feel safe driving for longer than twenty minutes. Plus, my impaired memory made it important for Mom to supplement my descriptions of symptoms and remind me what doctors said during appointments.

Dr. Two spent maybe ten minutes with me that day, despite a wait of over an hour. He reviewed the neurologist's report, said my condition sounded like it could be CFS, and said to keep taking the multivitamin and stimulant and to see him again in two months. I should've asked, "Why two months? What's going to change?" But no, I kept being the good, obedient little patient I'd been. I resolved to research some more conditions, though, now that I was done with school for the summer.

Each condition I discovered online was like a pinprick of light that I wanted to expand so that I could see if it was what I had. Multiple sclerosis. Sjögren's syndrome. Gilbert's syndrome. Benign adrenal tumor. Then, someone from church said my symptoms sounded like lupus, and I researched that. Crud, lupus was another possibility because its symptoms include prolonged fatigue, joint pain, and confusion. That summer, I quit my job at McDonald's after realizing working in a fast-paced, noisy environment that seemed to make me sicker wasn't worth the money. Even so, the job continued to disrupt my sleep in the form of something I have to this day that I call McNightmares. They're dreams about working overwhelmingly busy shifts where information such as buttons' locations keeps changing or where a procedure has changed so much that I don't know how to do it.

I went alone again to my July appointment because Mom had to work. The desire to know whether Dr. Two would diagnose me with CFS burned inside me. But after a wait of well over an hour, I was pretty sure that this would be my final visit with Dr. Two. After maybe five minutes in the room and a comment on my high blood pressure that day, he seemed ready to wrap up. He didn't care that I'd been waiting and waiting to learn something new about my condition from him. I was sweating to the point of embarrassment in the warm room, but I concentrated on the question I needed an answer for.

Unable to catch his eye as he scribbled out another prescription for the stimulant, I addressed the question to the top of his head, loudly: "So, do you think I have chronic fatigue syndrome?"

That made him look at my face but not my eyes. I'd had trouble sleeping the previous night because I'd been planning and rehearsing what to say, depending on his answer, in case my mind went blank. If he said yes, I would ask how I could learn to deal with it. If he said no, I would demand a hypothesis as to what I *did* have.

"I'm not sure yet," he responded with no emotion in his deep voice, as if I'd asked, "Do you think it's going to rain?"

No, no, no, that isn't right. I haven't planned a response to that! How can he look at me and say that?

As his eyes switched back to that darn scrip pad, I thought, *How dare you!* but managed to articulate, "Well, is there anything else we can do to help my fatigue? I'm still not functioning at 100 percent. I'm not sure I can go back to school like this."

"Fish oil," Dr. Two answered after a few seconds, looking confident, maybe even cheerful. "Fish oil supplements have been known to help with all sorts of health problems. I'll write you a prescription—what's in the over-the-counter supplements isn't always the same concentration. Take one a day. Let your dad try some, too. It might help with his stomach problems. Let me know if the copay is high." He was back to the scrip pad.

I'd heard of fish oil's multiple uses, but would it really help? I'd try it, of course. But I had to say more. I couldn't let him get away with writing a scrip to shut me up, and I did not want to leave until he addressed my concerns properly. I struggled to come up with the words to say.

"Mom's worried that I'll get worse. Well, moms do worry, I guess." Why I added the second sentence, I don't know, and I immediately regretted it.

"Yeah, I know. You'll be fine," he asserted while tucking his pen into his shirt pocket.

I was sure he did that to avoid meeting my eyes. It seemed dishonest to say I'd be fine, when he didn't know what was wrong. He seemed to think this statement would reassure me, but he didn't understand that I needed to know what was wrong.

When I told Mom and Dad about the appointment, they agreed that I needed a different doctor. I never pushed the fish oil on Dad, knowing it was a ridiculous suggestion for undiagnosed random vomiting episodes. Dad had an appointment with Dr. Two the next week, so he volunteered to get the form I needed to release my medical records. There was no showdown this time, just a two-week wait for the office staff to copy everything in my thickening file.

I learned another important lesson for patients: *trust yourself more than you trust health care professionals.* I try not to trust them at all. Sure, I respect their superior knowledge of medicine. Sure, I listen to what they say. However, regarding their words as absolute truth and their diagnoses as infallible can be hazardous to my health. I know my body better than any health care professional ever will because I'm the one living in it. I also thoroughly understand my experience with other forces that affect health, such as my emotional and spiritual well-being. Now, if I ever doubt something a physician tells me, I don't hesitate to express that doubt and then research symptoms and illnesses online or get a second opinion. Health care professionals are human and make mistakes because of lack of experience with certain conditions, bias or overconfidence, and stress, so I don't trust these people 100 percent. If I ever encounter another health care professional who has Dr. Two's combination of zeal for prescribing drugs and inability to listen actively, I'll leave immediately.

Another August arrived, the second one since my symptoms had started, and with it, commitment to another semester of being ill with no diagnosis. I searched online for patient reviews of local doctors. Doctors who sounded good didn't take our insurance or weren't affiliated with our hospital of choice. Come on, who wants to go to a hospital named *Hurley*, especially considering its proximity to rough Flint neighborhoods? My paternal grandmother, dead for a decade, had been a patient there once or twice and been disgusted by it. Her appraisal was probably accurate because she had made a living as a nurse. While reading reviews, I posted my reviews of Dr. One and Dr. Two to prevent other people from receiving inadequate care from them. My negative review of Dr. One joined that of another patient, who claimed that he'd made fun of her because of her mental illness.

Mom mentioned my search for a new doctor at work, and her boss with fibromyalgia urged us to try her doctor, who had diagnosed her condition after she'd spent months trying to determine the cause of her severe pain and exhaustion. She liked him as a person and a doctor. She described him as energetic, acting younger than his true age (late sixties). I had hoped for someone younger because I thought young doctors would be more familiar with current medical research, but she spoke so highly of this doctor that I laid aside my hesitation. Also, his clinic could do various blood tests and diagnostic imaging onsite. I liked that capability because it would save us time driving to other places for tests. So, I made an appointment with Dr. Three in late September.

My first impression was that Dr. Three was a man of action because he strode into the room so fast that the edges of his lab coat flapped like wings. With his shaved head and face, he didn't look his age. As I described my exhaustion, he reviewed my typed list of symptoms and illness timeline. I'd known I wouldn't be able to list all my symptoms and appointments with specialists on demand. Keeping in mind my previous experiences with doctors, I didn't let myself trust Dr. Three or hope that we'd find an answer that day.

"I go from doctor to doctor, specialist to specialist, but no one's figured out what's wrong," I explained. "My first doctor called me gaga."

"Pardon me?" Dr. Three asked, but his raised eyebrows showed he'd heard correctly. His glasses even slid down his nose somewhat.

"Gaga," I repeated.

"Crazy," Mom couldn't resist clarifying, and Dr. Three frowned.

Once I finished my story, he wrote something down, read a few pages from my records, mentioned my high blood pressure that day and on previous visits to Dr. Two, and agreed with me that it resulted from the stimulant. Then he said, "So, looking at these labs, you've had a lot of blood work done, but not much of any other kind of test. Blood tests are good for ruling out the common things. For instance, we know you're not anemic. But I think there's a few more things I can try, kiddo." He smiled.

First, he wanted to test the cortisol levels of my saliva. He explained that low cortisol levels signal a problem with the adrenal glands, which produce several important hormones. I'd researched conditions involving the adrenals before, and one of my many blood tests had measured cortisol. However, saliva testing was a more accurate way to assess cortisol levels, he said. He gave me a plastic bag with four vials in it. At four specific times in one day, I needed to spit enough to fill one three-milliliter vial. It wasn't the idea or action of spitting that grossed me out but the amount.

Also, he ordered some blood tests. He left the room, and a nurse/phlebotomist came in to take my blood. She had me sit in the chair next to Mom so that she could set the vials on the counter instead of on the examination table. After she finished, Mom and I were talking.

I stopped midsentence and said, "Mom, I don't feel good."

There was noise around me. I thought I'd fallen asleep because a trace of a dream involving a sunny, grassy hill floated in my mind's eye.

"What, what?" I asked. Oh, I'd fainted. I still didn't feel well. Someone in white lifted me off the chair and carried me to the examination table. I blinked and saw that it was Dr. Three. Only then did I notice the odor of smelling salts.

We never knew why I'd fainted because having blood drawn had never affected me. As unsettling as the experience was, I hoped that it would show Dr. Three that I was genuinely ill. Once we got home, we joked with Dad to keep him from worrying too much, saying the new doctor had swept me off my feet.

I had a dry mouth the next morning, so the first vial for the saliva test was the hardest to fill. I can't hawk and shoot spit, and for the first and only time ever, I wanted that ability. After about one minute of pushing saliva through my lips, they were sore. I resorted to putting a couple of drops of lemon juice on my tongue, as Dr. Three had said I could do if necessary. Staring at a chocolate dessert probably would've been as effective. The full process took a few minutes. I stuck the full vial in the fridge next to the butter, in plain sight so that I wouldn't forget where I'd put it.

About a week after I mailed the vials to the lab, Dr. Three's office called to arrange an appointment to discuss the test results. Knowing I wouldn't have been called if they had been normal, I was excited the rest of the week. I told my friends the results were apparently abnormal. At last, Friday came, and I drove home for the appointment.

When the time came, Dr. Three strode into the room and announced that my results were "pretty much normal." It was like he poured water over the little flame that had brightened my past few days. I could've sunk through the examination table and the floor. The normal finding should've been communicated over the phone so that I wouldn't have gotten the impression that my results were abnormal. My average cortisol level for the day was normal, which ruled out any gross malfunctioning of my adrenal glands. But the cortisol level was slightly below normal at 7 a.m. and 11 p.m. This indicated that some other process in my body was interfering somewhat with cortisol production.

Dr. Three admitted that he couldn't explain any further or guess what that other process could be. He said something about taking a different approach to diagnosing my illness.

He'd referred a patient with symptoms similar to mine to a homeopathic clinic, and a doctor there had figured out what was wrong with her and treated her. Dr. Three gave us the name of the clinic and the city it was in so that I could look it up online and think about going there. I felt open to trying a different kind of medicine. After all, the drugs and doctors I'd tried so far hadn't helped much. I felt a consuming letdown after the appointment and my return to campus.

Mom called the homeopathic clinic on Monday. When I listened to the voicemail message she left me afterward, I could hear in her greeting that something was wrong.

"There's a six-month waiting list," she continued. She'd scheduled an appointment for me there and sent in the required $300 deposit all the same.

I wanted to give up because six months of waiting sounded like forever. As I waited, I wondered about my future. I couldn't imagine my dreams of editing a best-selling book or traveling to Germany ever coming true. Once or twice, I wished that I had diabetes or cancer instead of whatever I did have, despite their severity, because they had treatments. I thought if I didn't improve soon, pursuing my degree would be pointless because of the damage it would do to my health and the unlikelihood of having a career. I reviewed the number of credits I needed for my English major and management minor and saw that I wouldn't be able to graduate in three and a half years as I had planned—and probably not even in four years.

Further interfering with my studies, my digestive problems worsened, causing episodes of indigestion and, worse, loose stool. I decided that I needed to do my own cooking so that I could have more control over what I ate and identify foods that triggered the problems. It wasn't possible to continue living in the dorms without a meal plan. So, I went through a stressful, drawn-out process to vacate my dorm room and cancel my meal plan at the end of the semester and find an apartment before the next one started. I would miss two of my roommates, the twins I'd befriended the previous school year. There was no chance I'd live with them the next school year. Helena would graduate in the spring, and Maria was getting an apartment for the next school year with her boyfriend (who became her husband after they graduated). My first request to cancel my dorm contract and meal plan was denied because I'd implied in my letter that the dining hall food was causing my digestive problems. I must've written that letter on one of those days when I had trouble writing complete sentences.

Mom and I met with the man who would make the decision concerning my second request. We took a copy of my medical records in case he didn't believe us when we said my undiagnosed condition was why I needed to live and cook independently. He listened to us without asking to see the papers and granted my request, even waiving the fee for breaking the dorm contract. That day, I also toured the unfurnished condo where I would live with four girls the next semester. My narrow bedroom had thin gray carpet and a closet without a door, probably because it was slightly narrower than the average door. Oh well, it was cheap and available.

While I was figuring out my living arrangements, there was good news and bad news. The good news was I could see the homeopathic doctor during the first week of 2011 because of a cancellation. The bad news was my night sweats were worsening. I was soaking my sheets, not just my pajamas, at least one night a week.

But on the first night of 2011, I had a thought that I wrote down in my journal and made a motto for myself: I don't know what the future holds, but I know God holds the future. I'm aware that a Google search of that sentence will return about a dozen results written by others who probably thought it before I did, but I don't recall having read it anywhere and would rather believe I was given that thought. I freely share it now so that it will provide others the same comfort it gave me.

CHAPTER THREE:
Supplements Fail to Lighten the Shadow
ଔ

Let's call this physician Dr. Nutrition. Although Dr. Three had called him a homeopathic doctor, his focus seemed to be nutrition. To get to Dr. Nutrition's clinic, where he and two other alternative medicine doctors practiced, we drove to a wealthy part of the state. He was tall and thin, and he had red hair. He talked with and examined me for forty-five minutes, even inspecting my tongue and fingernails.

"Hmm, you have ridges on your nails," he pointed out. "That indicates a nutrient deficiency."

This intrigued me. I'd considered studying nutrition as a minor in college and, even before I'd gotten sick, tried to eat well. That was one of the frustrations of being chronically ill: I'd taken such good care of myself that becoming so sick shouldn't have been possible—a flawed belief, yes, but one that many have.

He asked me what I ate and drank on a typical day.

"Whole-wheat bagel with low-fat cream cheese and a cup of coffee with Splenda or Equal for breakfast. A granola bar for a snack. A big salad with lite dressing and a glass of milk for lunch. Some chocolate, like two or three rows of a chocolate bar, for an afternoon snack. Dinner is something like a baked chicken breast, some steamed veggies, and mashed potatoes, with milk. I usually have some more chocolate after dinner," I rattled off.

"Not bad," he commented. "You shouldn't use Splenda or Equal. Use stevia. Splenda and Equal are unnatural and can upset your stomach. Stevia is natural and still tastes like sugar and has no calories. Now, about how much water are you drinking a day?"

"About one bottle."

"Mm, you need to drink at least twice that amount, okay? You need good hydration to have good health, and water flushes out toxins from your system."

After the examination, Dr. Nutrition prescribed several supplements that I could buy in the office and ordered blood tests to check for nutrient deficiencies, hormone imbalances, and food allergies. He also gave me a hair testing kit, explaining that this was another way to check for toxins in my system.

I left with a cloth tote bag of supplements and shock at how many hundreds of dollars the appointment and supplements had cost. The clinic took no insurance. According to Dr. Nutrition, that was because no insurance company wanted to cover natural treatments. There's such a stigma that treatments besides pharmaceutical products are useless or dangerous. As far as I could tell, all the supplements in that cloth bag were natural. One supplement was supposed to help with inflammation, and a powder supplement was supposed to boost energy. Not a single bottle came with a sheet of paper listing all the possible side effects, like you get with any prescription drug. I doubted that the supplements had half the potential to harm me that the drugs I'd tried, especially antidepressants, had.

For the rest of the month, I waited and wasn't surprised when I felt no more energetic. I'd known better than to get my hopes up. By not hoping that certain things would happen in high school, such as making it into advanced choirs, I'd avoided disappointment and been even happier after my accomplishments, and I'd applied that attitude to medical treatments. Although my digestion and trouble sleeping seemed slightly better, being back at school was still overwhelming. Many days, I wished that I'd withdrawn and felt, as I described it in my journal, "tired senseless." I regretted adding something to my plate that semester: becoming coeditor of a student publication. I'd taken it on because I'd thought this editing experience could compensate for not having completed an internship when I applied for editing jobs. Some days, I avoided calling Mom because I knew I'd start crying from exhaustion. We usually called or instant messaged each other every other day. I disliked making Mom and Dad worry about me because their worry accomplished nothing except making me feel guilty. I felt guilty when asking for help, so I usually didn't ask until one of my bad days, days on which the shadow was much heavier than usual.

Sometimes those days resulted from overexertion, but the ones without a cause were incredibly frustrating. I no longer had days when I felt better than usual.

The Friday before the third week of the semester, I had a bad day. I told Mom as we were instant messaging that I had papers due next week in both my German and human resource management classes on top of page-long responses to two classmates' stories for my fiction writing class. I couldn't do all those assignments. I hadn't had enough energy to read the stories or the next chapter in my biology textbook. I'd skipped biology again the previous day so that I'd have less walking and thinking to do.

"Is there something I can help with?" Mom typed.

At first, I thought of the dirty dishes I'd left in the sink—I didn't do dishes on bad days because I couldn't do them sitting down. Then I remembered all that homework. *Would it be right for her to help me with my homework?* A more attractive solution didn't present itself in the next minute, so I typed, "For those fiction responses, I have to write what I liked and what suggestions I have for improvement. If you could read the stories and tell me what you liked and didn't, that would save me time."

"You don't want me to write the actual reviews, do you?" she asked. She wasn't as confident in her writing skills as I was in mine.

"No, I'd better do that myself. Maybe you could send me bullet points of the good and bad things. I can get you the files I have to read now. I'd need the bullet points by Tuesday morning."

Mom did this task well enough to where I asked her to do the same thing another week. We agree on nearly everything, so she probably liked and disliked the same aspects of the stories that I would have. I didn't like asking her to contribute to my homework, considering I was secretary of an honor society that had integrity as one of its core values. Yes, I still had that office, having been unable to find a replacement at the start of the school year. I would've felt worse if I hadn't given my classmates the required feedback. In a few weeks, they would give me feedback on a story of my own, which I had yet to write.

While struggling with schoolwork, I'd pushed the latest blood tests to the back of my mind. They had to have been normal because I got no phone call indicating otherwise. I saw Dr. Nutrition again on February 1, and after greeting Mom and me, he told me I was deficient in pregnenolone, vitamin B_{12}, and potassium. My vitamin D and white blood cell counts were low. I was sensitive to gliadin and allergic to casein.

"Gliadin? Casein?" I asked.

"Gliadin means gluten, and casein means cow's milk, dairy," he answered. Dr. Nutrition told me to cut dairy from my diet and reduce my gluten intake. He explained that a full gluten-free diet means no oats, wheat, barley, or rye and gave me a packet listing products and foods in which gluten is a hidden ingredient.

I tried to process Dr. Nutrition's findings as Mom and I got into our car.

"Let's go to that Whole Foods we saw on the way here," Mom suggested. "They should have dairy-free and gluten-free stuff." We'd never been to a Whole Foods Market before.

I agreed, and as we pulled out of the clinic's parking lot, I thought aloud, "I wonder why none of the other doctors thought to test for food allergies. I drink two glasses of milk a day, so no wonder I'm having digestive problems. Not to mention all the chocolate." *Chocolate*. My shoulders slumped as I chewed on the thought that I couldn't eat my favorite food.

Mom, knowing my thoughts, said, "You could probably eat dark chocolate."

"No," I answered. "I want to get better. I won't risk taking even one bite of dairy." As disappointed as I was in my previous doctors for not catching the obvious problem of an allergy to dairy, I was glad I could do something to feel better quickly. I started drinking soymilk that afternoon.

I was thankful Dr. Nutrition said I could wean off the two ineffective supplements he had prescribed last time, because now I had to take pregnenolone (a building block of steroid hormones), magnesium, vitamin B_{12}, and vitamin D. When I took my last dose of the powdered energy supplement Sunday before I returned to school, I reread the label on the container before throwing it away and saw *D-Ribose* printed below the brand name. That word sounded familiar. Maybe it had been a treatment for some disorder I'd researched online.

Mom cooked all weekend long to help me begin my diet. One of the first dairy- and gluten-free recipes Mom made was brownies, despite my new fear that chocolate would harm me. By Sunday evening, she'd filled a box full of meals I could eat. After my twin friends and I finished the brownies, in ten days I lost the five pounds I'd gained during Christmas vacation, because I wasn't snacking on chocolate daily. No other sweet was good enough to replace it. I hadn't thought I was addicted to chocolate, but depriving myself of it gave me a taste of what trying to beat addiction is like. I craved it and felt sad when I passed it in the grocery store. Grocery shopping became time-consuming, draining, and expensive. Well, it had already been draining because of the stimulation from all the colored labels and varieties of food, all the shoppers, and all the music playing, on top of pushing a cart and calculating which brand of cereal was the cheapest that day. Now I also had to read food labels carefully. Case in point: Mom and I had bought a box of chocolate chip cookies labeled *nondairy* at Whole Foods, but when I read the ingredients list before eating them, it declared, "Contains less than 2 percent of the following: milk." That's not nondairy! How did the company get away with labeling the box *nondairy*? I didn't eat much meat, so finding foods with good amounts of protein and fiber was necessary so that I wouldn't feel as ravenous as I'd felt so far. The twins bought me a dairy-free chocolate bar, but it tasted like wax.

I wasn't looking forward to Valentine's Day, which for me is Eat Extra Chocolate Day. I've always been single, and I don't plan to marry. One bad day before the holiday, I felt dejected and miserably bushed to the point where I was tempted to skip church, which Mom and I do only when traveling. A contributor to my mood that morning was that Grampa had won his battle with colon cancer by going to heaven the week before, and I felt bad for not being able to attend his funeral with my parents. Traveling and then doing makeup work would've been too overwhelming. Plus, my plane tickets to and from Wyoming would've cost as much as three months of rent. At church, I heard what would have been an uplifting sermon if I had been concentrating more on Pastor's words than on not crying. I resolved to stop at Walgreen's on the way back to my apartment. I'd buy green tea to warm and maybe wake me and a chocolate bar with as little dairy as possible. I didn't care if my stomach didn't like it later. I needed *something* to cheer me up now.

I read the allergy information of chocolate bar after chocolate bar. Finally, I found a Lindt 70 percent cacao bar whose label said "May contain traces of dairy." *May. Traces.* That would work! I turned to go check out, and perfect words came over the radio: words about lifting burdens and not giving up.

Josh Groban, my favorite singer, was singing "You Are Loved (Don't Give Up)" straight to me. I'd heard the song only once before. If you've never heard his voice, imagine a rich baritone, gently warbling, that makes you feel like you're sinking into a hot bath. I smiled and knew that not only was Josh singing to me, but God was singing also. God had planned this moment for me with the care taken to plan a marriage proposal or surprise party. I stood still, filled with awe at being singled out, chin high, unconscious of others in the store, listening to the next verse, which had words about hidden hurt and feeling lost.

The decadent chocolate I ate after lunch was the best I'd ever tasted. Better yet, the next day, a package from a dairy-free food company arrived. It contained five dairy-free chocolate bars that tasted as rich as the Lindt bar. It was a Valentine's Day gift from my parents.

In late March, it was time to register for summer and fall classes. I wanted to take a break over the summer, and I clearly couldn't take four classes in the fall semester. I chose three. First was an English course on Detroit publishers. The industrial/organizational psychology course I wanted to take was offered online, so I chose that option to avoid exerting myself getting to campus for it. The third class would require exertion, though, because it was a graduate-level editing course that ran from 7 to 9:50 p.m. one night a week. I've never been a night owl, so concentrating during that class would've been tough even if I'd been healthy.

"Now, there's one problem with taking just three classes," I explained to my friend Helena. "That's considered part-time. My remaining scholarships require me to attend full-time, so I'm going to lose them." That sacrifice would cost $4,000.

"Oh, that stinks," she said.

"I know. Scholarships have paid for about a third of my costs."

"Will you still work at the Writing Center?" she asked.

"Yeah. I don't want to quit because I like it so much, and I'm getting experience that will be good for editing. How much good will a degree do without experience?"

After our conversation, I thought about appealing the loss of my scholarships because a disability, not laziness, had made me reduce my course load, but I lacked the energy to fight it. No wonder people with disabilities are disadvantaged in life: self-care takes too much energy and time for us to act to get fair treatment. Plus, thanks to medical expenses, we can't afford to invest as much in stocks or bonds, buy as many tools and resources, or sue in response to gross injustice. I'd begun referring to my health problems as a disability sometimes when talking to those I was close with. Just because what I had was undiagnosed and invisible to others didn't mean it wasn't disabling.

This perspective came from befriending Beth, a coworker who used a wheelchair. Her hair was light brown and wavy, usually in a ponytail. Like me, she had blue eyes, wore glasses, and was a bit nerdy about grammar. She was one of the most cheerful people I'd met, and she had a contagious smile perfect for a toothpaste commercial. Beth was working on her master's degree in English, having earned her bachelor's in neuroscience. In the past six months, we'd shared our frustrations: mine with my doctors and my lack of a diagnosis and hers with the only somewhat reasonable accommodations Central Michigan University had provided.

One day, I felt bold enough to ask why she used a wheelchair. I was sure she didn't want to be characterized as "the girl in the wheelchair" just as I didn't want to be characterized as "the girl who's tired all the time." Even so, I was curious. Beth and I were toward the back of the library Writing Center location, out of earshot of everyone else. Beth was online but on a website that didn't appear to have anything to do with work. She made an irritated sound twice in one minute, so I asked what was wrong. Beth complained about her health insurance. The company didn't want to pay for a modification to her wheelchair that would make maneuvering in winter easier. It argued that the modification was unnecessary for mobility because it was seasonal. Both of us had experienced the tendency for health insurance to fight us. She told me part of the reason for the conflict between the company and her was that her condition had an unpredictable course.

"May I ask what you have?" I asked quietly.

"It's called Friedreich's ataxia," she answered in her very soft voice, explaining that it's a progressive degenerative neurological disorder. It sounded kind of like muscular dystrophy. She was gradually losing her ability to control her movements, and even worse, there was no treatment and no cure.

Wow. For a few seconds, I gazed at the watercolor of a peacock hanging on the wall above Beth's computer, wanting to say something comforting. The best I could come up with was "At least you have a diagnosis. You know what's happening. I, well, it would be nice to have some idea of what I have."

"I can understand that," Beth said gently. "That's hard. For a while, I didn't know what I had. A neurologist found out what it was."

A couple of days later, the implication of "progressive degenerative" sank in. The illness or a complication of it would eventually take her life. Compared with what she was going through, why was I letting my health problems bother me so much, making me smile less and complain more to God?

My complaining increased when my digestive symptoms, after a month of improvement, intensified. Stomachaches gave way to loose stool, gas, and more pain. By *loose stool*, I mean something slightly better than diarrhea: small blobs that were sometimes hard to pass and even harder to know when they were all out. Oh, all right, I'll say what I mean to ease the embarrassment others with this problem have: I experienced incontinence. I recorded everything I ate for two weeks, trying to figure out which food or food group was causing the problems. I reread the ingredients of every food product I had to ensure that I wasn't eating dairy.

I wondered whether I was absorbing the dozen or so tablets I now took daily. Somehow, I managed to keep straight which supplements to take when. I resisted buying a pill sorter because that seemed like something for old people, not me. Instead, I lined up the bottles in a cupboard in the same order at home and my apartment. I put the supplements I took three times a day on one side and the supplements I took twice a day on the other.

In April, I had loose stool three times in eight days. Despite not wanting to wear myself out worse by driving home, I went to see Dr. Three. I felt no pain when he pressed on my abdomen, but he could hear the ominous gurgling signaling that another episode of loose stool was coming. He told me to cut all gluten from my diet, prescribed an antibiotic in case there was an infection, and ordered a stool test. The test—surprise, surprise—came back normal, meaning no obvious blood or infectious agent was in my stool. He also referred me to an allergist to see if food allergies were causing my digestive trouble, and I set the appointment for June because I couldn't keep interrupting my busy semester with appointments.

I was worn out and worn in, worn down and worn up, despite not putting my full effort into my classes, despite skipping one ten times. I would've sacrificed one of my scholarships if I'd let my grade point average drop below 3.5, so I couldn't be a complete slacker. Looking at everything I had to do in my planner was discouraging because I added more than what I subtracted from the list. Sometimes I forgot to do assignments even when I wrote them down. I judged that my functioning was down to 50 percent of my pre-illness level. I no longer power walked to and from classes. My muscly shoulders from four years of high school swimming, my favorite part of my body, were dissolving into shadow. I could barely do push-ups, on those rare days when I could force myself to do them, because of a sharp pain in my right wrist whenever I put weight on it. I had little energy to clean the apartment, and my roommates didn't seem to care about cleaning. I knew an unclean environment could harm my health more.

Embarrassed and guilty but desperate, I asked Mom to help me clean the kitchen when she and Dad visited me on Easter. She insisted on doing it herself, so while she cleaned, I sat outside with Dad as he grilled chicken. Easter came so late that year that outdoor cooking was possible.

"Your mom said you're not taking any classes this summer," he said, frowning.

I knew he wanted to know why I wasn't. I'd taken one online class every summer I'd been in college. "I need a break," I explained while thinking, *I want to give up on school.* I was afraid of how he'd react if I said that, though. "This semester has been really rough, especially with the digestive problems. I just can't do as much anymore. I *will* work at the Writing Center this summer, at least ten hours a week. I should know the exact number soon." It would be the most hours per week I'd ever worked there. My supervisors had kindly accommodated my needs ever since I had told them the previous year why I couldn't work more.

He nodded, but I wasn't sure that he was satisfied. I didn't know how to make him understand how much my condition had worsened that semester. He often forgot things I told him about school, thanks to the memory loss that accompanies middle age. As Dad flipped the chicken, I reminded myself that I would graduate in December of the following year. If I quit now, I probably would never go back. I needed my degree to get a decent, doable job. Without a diagnosis, getting federal disability benefits, my alternative to working, appeared impossible. Besides, I'd heard that going on disability was more trouble than it was worth.

During the last weeks of the semester, with both gluten and dairy out of my diet and a limited budget for special gluten-free products, I stressed out about what to eat. I even replaced half my food with soymilk and fruit juice. Besides, I didn't want to eat if the food would end up being the slimy lumps I kept passing. The only foods that seemed safe were popcorn and mixed vegetables, which became my dinner on several evenings. Oh well, that was simple to cook. I was probably consuming trace amounts of gluten by sharing a kitchen with four women, but I didn't understand why my digestion continued to deteriorate.

I had less and less time for homework as I spent more and more time on the toilet and in the shower because I couldn't stand being unclean after passing loose stool. I wished I could've vomited instead because that would've been quicker. The antibiotic Dr. Three had prescribed didn't help. Pepto Bismol could alleviate any remaining pain after an episode but couldn't prevent recurrences. I decreased the amount of magnesium I was taking because I'd read somewhere that too much of it could work like a laxative. I considered buying disposable underwear to wear in case I lost control away from the apartment, but I felt too embarrassed to buy some and made do with panty liners. Sleep didn't always offer an escape from worries about my bowels because I often had nightmares about having accidents all over the bathroom floor, nightmares that return occasionally now.

My top ribs were as visible as they had been during my senior-year swim team days, when I had weighed about 113 pounds and owned a pair of size one jeans. It was too bad that I'd gotten rid of those jeans, because I now walked with an elbow or a textbook pressed to one hip out of fear that my pants would fall down. I was hungry and frustrated.

Frustrated was another word that, like *tired* and *exhausted*, I now disliked because I wrote and spoke it so often. I started slipping into dark thoughts again, such as *What good is my life, if I have to spend it like this? I can't tolerate this life. I don't want to care about anything because of the energy it requires. I want to go home!* One night, I wrote this in my journal: "Mentally, I am in fetal position." I arranged to get counseling over the summer to help me deal with the stress of living like this in a healthier way.

A couple of weeks later, I had loose stool three times in eight days again. This episode came with weakness and extra exhaustion for a few days afterward. The worsened digestion baffled Dr. Nutrition. I ran the old idea that I had chronic fatigue syndrome by him. He said maybe we could call it that, but doing so wouldn't be very useful because it had no treatment. I accepted that statement as true, too bushed to ask any follow-up questions. He drew blood to check for autoimmune disease markers.

When the test results came back as normal, he prescribed a supplement to take with aloe juice. He said if this didn't help, there was nothing more he could do for me. He didn't offer to refer me to either of his colleagues, so I assumed that they also couldn't help. After trying the last supplement and soapy-tasting aloe juice grudgingly for a month, wondering whether he'd simply wanted to get a little more money out of us, I weaned off my ineffective supplements, including the new one. To this day, I have the ridges on my fingernails that he pointed out to me. Maybe I've always had them, and maybe they mean nothing.

CHAPTER FOUR:
Naming the Shadow
☙

Ready to try something else, I saw Dr. Three again in May. Hypoparathyroidism—a mouthful meaning that a structure within the thyroid isn't working right—was the latest possible diagnosis I'd heard about from someone at church and researched online. Symptoms included fatigue, muscle twitches, and muscle spasms. After hearing my concern about hypoparathyroidism, Dr. Three ordered a thyroid ultrasound, surprised I hadn't had one done already. The test came back, as Dr. Three put it, "extraordinarily normal," and as I put it, "exasperatingly normal."

After the semester ended, I resumed counseling for six weeks to help me deal with my stress and the guilt I felt for making my parents work harder to assist me. With my counselor's guidance, I accepted the new career plan as a freelance editor or writing tutor, working from home instead of my dream city of Chicago, that I'd developed over the past year. Clearly, I couldn't work outside the home and full-time in this condition, so freelancing seemed like the best way to do what I enjoyed and had shown aptitude for and to make a reasonable income. Maybe I could do something productive with my life after all. Also, the counselor helped me correct some patterns of negative thinking I'd developed.

"That's false guilt," she said when I described feeling bad for asking for my parents' help.

What do you mean, "false"? I really feel this way, I thought.

"Asking for help is not a sin," the counselor explained. "You know the Ten Commandments. That's not one of them. There are times when we all have to ask for help. That's not wrong, so there's no reason to feel guilt." She soon convinced me that being unable to function fully on my own was acceptable, but she had to tell me more to reduce the negative feeling's power.

"You didn't bring this illness on yourself," she brought out at one point. "It's not like you were abusing drugs and that caused your illness. You took care of yourself, it sounds like. This isn't your fault."

I got into the habit of reminding myself often that Mom and Dad were willing to make their sacrifices out of love for me and willing to assist me if it eased the suffering they saw. One of several helpful activities my counselor recommended was watching a new movie called *Soul Surfer*. It's about Bethany Hamilton, a professional surfer who at age fourteen lost an arm after a shark attack and, with her Christian faith and family's support, made a magnificent comeback to surfing. The part that stood out the most to me came toward the end, when footage from a real interview with

Hamilton appeared. A journalist asked her whether she would've gone surfing on the day of the attack if she had known beforehand what would happen. Hamilton answered that she wouldn't have changed what happened and that she has been able to embrace more people with one arm than she had with two.

The movie encouraged me to make the most of, or at least something good of, my life despite my illness. A loss of health doesn't equal a loss of life. Even if I were to lose all my physical abilities, I'd find a way to express myself and love to family and friends. I hope other patients with chronic illnesses learn this faster than I. Positive thinking certainly isn't a cure or even a treatment for ailments, but good emotional health makes dealing with poor physical health easier. Being positive doesn't mean skipping through sunny days with a cheesy grin. To me, it means being skeptical of the future by remembering that life could get better instead of worse, even while having plans in place in case my health declines.

A second constructive activity built on one I'd done since a conversation with my friend Maria the previous semester: writing three positive thoughts about my day or life in my journal every night. My counselor had me add one negative thought nagging me and then put a positive spin on it or ask myself whether this thought would matter a year from now. For example, I wrote, "I miss Mom, *but* going home this weekend would've used up time and kept me from catching up on cleaning here." I'd moved into a different apartment in May and was living there with plenty of spiders and dust bunnies. My two assigned roommates would arrive in August. This place was an improvement over the condo where I'd lived the previous semester. It had a little patio, was furnished with wood and metal tables and chairs that matched anything, and had no stairs. My bedroom and closet were as big as the ones I had at home.

I faced a challenge to my more positive attitude when a new symptom began in June. At first, I thought it was a rash on my face. But as it emerged on my chest, upper arms, neck, and back, I examined it, discovering it was acne, the worst acne I'd ever had. Each new spot took about a month to fade. I tried several over-the-counter creams and diluted tea tree oil, a natural remedy I'd found online, but none worked. Suddenly, I looked fifteen instead of twenty-one. I'd always been thankful that my illness hadn't affected my appearance or made people stare at me. Now my appearance had changed so much that for the first time, I wanted to wear makeup besides lip gloss and was embarrassed to be seen in a swimsuit.

An invisible problem persisted that summer, too. My wrist still hurt whenever I bent my hand back or put weight on it, so much so that I had it examined and x-rayed at the campus clinic. There was no sign of a fracture or of carpal tunnel syndrome, so the doctor gave me a brace to wear and an anti-inflammatory medicine. For a week after that appointment, I was more enervated than usual. Finally, I suspected the medicine was behind the increased exhaustion, so I stopped taking it. Living with the pain was easier than having decreased ability to function. With time, the pain became a weekly rather than daily occurrence.

By the middle of June, I'd cheated on my gluten-free, dairy-free diet a few times out of frustration; my attitude was that I had problems, no matter what I ate. Surprisingly, I digested forbidden crackers painlessly. My appointment with the allergist was that month. I told her about all my symptoms and how the digestive ones had intensified when I had stopped eating gluten. She said the worsened digestion indicated that gluten wasn't the source of my problems. She ordered skin scratch tests for every kind of grain, dairy, and chocolate. *Skin scratch* is too gentle a name. The tests involved a nurse inserting food derivatives just under my skin, which felt like she was using a stapler down my back. Nearly every puncture made me flinch. When the nurse finished, she said not to touch my back. We waited to see if I'd have any reaction, but none of the spots itched or swelled. The allergist examined them and declared I had no food allergies, to my delight.

I thought that would end the appointment. But she read on one of the forms I'd filled out that I was allergic to ragweed and cats, so she tested me for various environmental allergies. A different nurse did the skin scratching this time. To my surprise, none of the new puncture spots itched, though I knew the allergist had included ragweed and cats in the list of allergens to test. When the allergist returned to examine the spots, the nurse handed her a paper that I assumed was the list.

"But we already did those," the allergist said. "These food ones—we already did them. You were supposed to do the other tests, the environmental ones." She flipped the nurse's file folder open. "Yes. See this sheet here?"

"Oh. Oh, I'm sorry," the nurse said. Anger flashed through me.

"Just one moment," the allergist said to Mom and me, and she and the nurse left the room.

I hoped the allergist was having stern words with that nurse. I was lying on my stomach, with my head facing away from Mom, so I couldn't see her reaction. But without her saying a word, I knew she was more upset than I.

Counseling was making it easier to find and focus on positives in life. The only positive I could see in this situation was that we could be certain I had no food allergies because I'd had those tests twice. The nurse returned a minute later with sincere apologies for her mistake. Even so, I didn't look forward to having even more spots jabbed. There wasn't much undisturbed skin left on my poor back, so some of the new spots were on the back of my left arm. Some of them itched—a lot. I wanted the allergist to come in to examine me *now*. After what seemed like far too long, she returned. She told me I was allergic to ragweed, cats, one kind of grass, one kind of tree, and dust mites and mildly allergic to dogs.

The appointment had taken so long that going out for dessert to celebrate my lack of food allergies would have spoiled our appetite for dinner, but I ate plenty of chocolate and pasta in the next week. I still drank soymilk, preferring its taste and longer shelf life and preferring not to wonder about dairy cows' living conditions and what steroids they were given. Also, I still consumed very little cheese because it seemed Dr. Nutrition's blood test must've shown an allergy to dairy for some reason. My diet changes decreased my loose stools to monthly rather than weekly occurrences but failed to generate more energy.

Dr. Three now seemed out of ideas, and I wanted more advanced care. In the summer of 2011, Dr. Three's office made an appointment with an internist at the University of Michigan (U of M) Health System, now called Michigan Medicine. After conducting a physical and listening to my description of symptoms, she referred me to an endocrinologist and a rheumatologist and coordinated the care I received from the system. Having seen one endocrinologist, I had some idea of that specialty's focus but was curious enough about how it might view my exhaustion to borrow an endocrinology textbook from the library and learn about hormones and glands. I didn't know what rheumatology was, so I turned to an online medical dictionary, which said rheumatologists specialize in conditions like arthritis and are interested in unexplained fatigue, weight loss, weakness, muscle or joint pain, and anemia. Knowing that, I wondered why I hadn't seen a rheumatologist earlier. Of course, I had to wait to see the doctors.

While I waited, I started writing about everything that was happening to me. I kept thinking others shouldn't experience what I was going through with having no diagnosis, with doctors who didn't know or do enough, and with struggling in school. Writing felt like doing something positive with these negative experiences, which was slightly comforting. Plus, if I didn't write my experiences down, I would forget them, as poor as my memory was. I wrote an essay, titled "Sinking Self-Image," about one facet of my struggles.

Here is a shortened version of that essay:

Learning to live with a chronic illness has presented challenges of various sizes and shapes. My self-image has certainly taken a dunking, and living with the result is a minor challenge among the many I face because of this illness. But when I think of how rarely I swim now, or when I look in the mirror, thoughts about my self-image sometimes surface from deep inside. I miss the self-image and physical appearance I had at age eighteen. A picture of me at the high-school swimming conference championship epitomizes how I looked and felt about myself then.

My favorite feature in the picture is my shoulders. They stand out because I'm stretching my arms with my fingers entwined at the crown of my head, which is covered by my black team cap. Even though the photo is somewhat blurry, I can see biceps, triceps, and other muscles whose names I don't know. My shoulders are definitely wider than my hips, not that my hips are wide. It took lots of laps to get those dangerous-looking shoulders.

I have no flab anywhere, not even on my stubborn thighs. My hands could almost encircle my waist. Yes, I was thin—too thin, in Mom's eyes. I stand behind a starting block, goggles on. My swimsuit is red and black, in a pattern that looks like fireworks. I look great in it, if I may say so. I'm smiling, looking toward my left, maybe at a teammate in Lane 3. I look ready to go take fifth in the conference in the 200-yard freestyle.

And now? It's been months since I've swum, and that red-and-black swimsuit is taking up space in a drawer. My favorite feature is still my shoulders, which I've fought to keep respectable but no longer look tough. There's a smaller difference between my shoulders' and hips' widths. I don't feel tough or strong, well, not physically. Emotionally, mentally, I've grown stronger. That part of my self-image isn't struggling to swim.

Even more important, my faith and relationship with Jesus Christ are stronger. What I've lost in physical strength, I've gained in spiritual strength. And what keeps me from sinking in a pool of self-pity is remembering which kind of strength is most important. I'd rather have that strength than awe-inspiring muscles.

As I continued to wait for my two appointments at the U of M, a bill for nearly $800 came from the allergist's office. My insurance had covered nothing. I thought there must've been a mistake. I'd given Mom's insurance card to the receptionist and asked whether we owed anything before we left. No one had said anything to suggest that my insurance wouldn't cover the appointment and tests in full. I didn't understand everything about my insurance plan—who does?

My irritation with the clinic increased when I called the allergist's office manager, who obviously didn't understand insurance policies any more than I did. Now that my parents had to pay this big bill, I was upset that the allergist had bothered testing for allergies to ragweed and cats, when my symptoms had been strong enough evidence. After not getting sympathy or help from the clinic, I tried calling my insurance company. It turned out our plan covered no allergy care, period. Why it didn't cover allergies when it covered just about everything else, I didn't know. It's not like allergies are trivial ailments. They can kill people. Despite how upset I was with the lack of insurance coverage and the unethical actions of the allergist's office, my parents paid the bill.

When I finally saw the two specialists, they joined my growing list of doctors who were unable to shed light on my illness. The endocrinologist was more interested in my polycystic ovary syndrome than in my mysterious exhaustion. She had me try going off my birth control pills and trying a different brand three months later. That medicine caused periods that lasted for two weeks with much cramping beforehand. The other medicines we tried over the course of a year, after which I gave up on her, caused problems that included soreness, nausea, and depression. Remembering my previous intolerance of antidepressants and of the anti-inflammatory, it dawned on me that I had another symptom: sensitivity to medications.

The rheumatologist prescribed nothing but frustrated me in her own way. She examined my hands and feet and confirmed a diagnosis of Raynaud's disease I'd received that winter from Dr. Three. Raynaud's disease is a condition in which the smallest blood vessels in the hands and feet overreact to temperature change. It causes abnormally cold hands or feet and color changes in them. I didn't think the Raynaud's was related to my current illness because I'd had poor circulation since my early teens. She continued her examination, finding nothing abnormal.

"Any idea what's wrong with me?" I asked. "The only thing I can think of is chronic fatigue syndrome."

"I wouldn't diagnose you with chronic fatigue syndrome," the rheumatologist answered in what I guessed was an eastern European accent.

Does she mean that she doesn't think I have it or that she wouldn't diagnose anyone with it?

Before I could ask, she added, "You need to think positive. That's quite helpful. I see patients with much worse conditions. I know you're taking an antidepressant, but you might want additional therapy, if anxiety is an issue. Be positive."

I nodded, expecting her to add something more meaningful.

"Well, of course it's good to be positive, but she's really sick!" Mom exclaimed. "That's not going to cure her. Before she got sick, she was taking eighteen credits and working three jobs. Now, she can hardly do her homework, let alone have a job. There's something *wrong*." (She told me later she wanted to add, "Come here so I can slap you!")

I didn't want the doctor to be upset. Seeing Mom angry was startling because that's a rare emotion for her. But she was right, except I'd had two jobs, not three.

"I'm just talking to my patient," the rheumatologist countered, a hand in front of her in defense. "I'm just telling you what I think is best. And you should encourage her. Stressing her out will not help her. Encouragement *will* help."

She thought for a few moments. "If your sleep isn't refreshing"—I nodded—"then perhaps you should go to our sleep clinic. The U of M has an excellent sleep clinic. There might be something interfering with your sleep. I can refer you to them."

I doubted that a sleep study would find anything. I don't snore. Mom had heard me talk in my sleep and had discovered my other quirky sleep characteristic when one time she found me sleeping with my eyes open, making her panic because she thought I was dead. Anyway, another part of me knew that I was running out of possible diagnoses. I was among the best doctors in the state, so if I had some unusual disease, they were the most likely candidates to discover it. I perceived a chance that I had CFS, but if my case bewildered these specialists, how could I possibly make a diagnosis? Plus, if I had that, then I would be stuck like this forever. Done. Disabled. Because of these thoughts and unwillingness to resign myself to lifelong disability, I had the rheumatologist refer me to the sleep clinic.

I suppose that I was a frustrating patient for her. As my friend Beth reminded me when I told her about this appointment, doctors are used to being able to figure out what's wrong with someone. They have extensive training. But I wished that the rheumatologist had known how frustrating it was for me to hear "I don't know" from yet another medical professional and for me to live like this. She, like all the other doctors I'd seen, couldn't believe that I was seriously ill because I had no visible signs of illness. No, I wasn't sneezing blue snot or growing a third arm. No, my labs weren't often abnormal. But doctors, please understand that if all your technology shows that nothing is wrong with patients, there may still be something very wrong with them, and the malady isn't necessarily psychological.

I'm not the only one who has had these thoughts after frustrating encounters with doctors. In a book I read a few years after this appointment, *Encounters with the Invisible*, Dorothy Wall writes that it's wrong for doctors to have the simple view that illnesses with visible pathology are the only ones that exist. Illness is a subjective experience that objective science may be unable to measure conclusively. Health care professionals should use medical technology alongside of, not as a replacement for, their brains and what patients say they feel, explains Wall, who has a chronic illness. For example, I think doctors rely too much on what laboratories say is the normal range for blood tests. Granted, I don't know how those normal ranges were decided on, but what if a level of a chemical, hormone, or type of blood cell that's normal for one person results in symptoms for another? What if people with some chronic illnesses need higher blood concentrations of specific nutrients or hormones to be in optimal health?

Despite my skepticism about doctors and the sleep study, I returned to the U of M that August. The U of M does sleep studies in two parts. First, patients have an appointment with a sleep medicine specialist. Then, if the specialist thinks having an overnight study would be insightful, he or she orders one. The specialist examined my ears, nose, and throat; listened to my chest; and talked with me about my sleep habits, the annoying sinuses I'd inherited from Mom, and the content of my dreams and nightmares (usually that my parents are mad at or disowning me). Afterward, she was uncertain whether I should have an overnight study.

She was sure that I didn't have common sleep disorders, like restless legs syndrome or sleep apnea. However, she explained that there was a small chance I had a rare and infrequently detected kind of sleep apnea called upper airway resistance. Patients with that disorder usually don't snore and usually are thin, which were two characteristics I had. The U of M was one of a handful of places in the country that could test for upper airway resistance. She let me decide whether I should have a sleep study. I scheduled one, adding my name to the two-month-long waiting list. I suspected that this would be another fruitless test but was so desperate for a diagnosis that I couldn't pass on this opportunity.

The opportunity came just two weeks later, thanks to a cancellation. The test for upper airway resistance involved threading a tiny tube, probably half the diameter of a straw, up my nose, down my esophagus, and into my chest cavity. This was in addition to all the other wires and electrodes glued all over me, from the top of my head to my feet. The sleep test technician had a hard time getting the tube in.

"It's like there's a brick wall at the back of your nose," he said after his third attempt, looking puzzled. He shook his dreads back from his face. "Why would you put a brick wall in your nose?"

I grimaced, assured him that I hadn't been the one to put the wall in my nose, and eased my death grip on the chair, having been told earlier that relaxing made the insertion easier. Thankfully, he and another technician were able to force the tube up my other nostril. I hadn't wanted the tube to go in that nostril because the sleep medicine specialist had found—stop reading this paragraph if you gross out easily—a polyp in there. Both my grandpas had died from colon cancer, making me think of cancer first when I heard her say *polyp*, but it's completely benign, simply a slight blockage. The tube insertion process didn't hurt, but I felt every part of it and gagged when the tube scooted down my throat. Then, I was supposed to sleep somehow, after going through such a weird ordeal.

The technicians left to test their monitoring equipment in another room. I lay down, said something to Mom, and felt the tube in my throat when I spoke. I wanted to clear my throat or cough, but I assumed that would interfere with the measurements.

"I can feel the tube . . . when I talk," I told her softly.

"Then don't talk," she replied matter-of-factly. We looked at each other for a few moments. She knew what I was thinking: I didn't like this situation at all and didn't want to move for fear of dislodging any wires. She rose from the smaller-than-twin foldout bed next to my large hospital bed, bent over me, slid her hands under my shoulder blades in an awkward but much-needed hug, and kissed my cheek. I remember receiving only two other kisses from Mom in my life because we prefer hugging. Some things are better said with hugs.

"Thank you," I whispered.

"You look so miserable," Mom said, and the sadness shadowing her face must have mirrored mine.

I probably looked like a cross between a robot and Frankenstein's monster. Mom shouldn't have had to see me like this. She'd always dismissed my apologies for putting her through everything my illness was putting her through. She'd never griped about having to drive me anywhere or do chores I'd once helped her with. I'd willingly helped her around the house since age two, according to my baby book. I was sick of subjecting us to all these tests, so I prayed this one would find something. It took almost an hour to fall asleep after the lights went off. I remember changing positions, very slowly, three times, finally ending up on my stomach, ignoring the tension in my right cheek as the medical tape strained to hold the electrode there.

Over breakfast the next morning, Mom and I shared our thoughts. Given the difficulty with the tube, the possibility of some upper airway resistance or sinus problem messing with my sleep seemed more real. Plus, Mom told me she'd seen a shooting star the night before my study. Although we don't believe in wishing on stars, she'd felt like that star meant something good. I started the fall semester a few days later with hope growing in me like a vine. Maybe I could still have a normal life and career that served God. Maybe I could finally figure out what was casting that oppressive shadow.

I got a phone call from Dad one evening about a week after the study. He said the sleep specialist had called, and I was surprised to hear an upset tone.

"She said there was no sleep . . . app-nee-uh. Apnea," Dad said slowly, obviously reading from phonetically spelled notes he'd taken while on the phone. "No resistance or . . . breathing problem. Everything was normal."

"Normal? Really?" I asked. Neither of us was sure what to say. I tried to think about something besides the shock. "Well, I guess I can cancel the follow-up appointment with her," I said stiffly.

"Yeah, I guess. Mom's playing volleyball tonight, but I'll, uh, I'll let her know about this."

"I guess I've got to figure out what to try next." I sighed. "I don't know. I'll think of something." We didn't say much more. I felt tears coming as I set my phone down.

I had no hope, no idea what to do now. *Why are you letting this happen to me, God?* I sat on my bed and let the tears loose. Holding them in seemed like a poor way to spend the energy I had left. I wanted Mom but refused to call her and interrupt her evening of fun with her team. *I can't take this. How is this going to be good for me?* I was thinking of a usually comforting Bible verse I'd memorized from the text framed in my bedroom: "For I know the plans I have for you . . . plans to give you hope and a future" (Jeremiah 29:11). I felt my frustration transforming into anger at God. I knew I'd regret that anger later, so I tried a different tack.

I grabbed the box of tissues out of the bathroom, blew my nose, and grabbed my journal to vent in by writing all the questions I wanted answered. My head felt pressurized from trying to control my crying and streaming snot. I asked whether God really was perfect, really cared about me, and really would help me through this. I knew I sure didn't deserve his help, seeing as I was doubting and criticizing him in my wondering and writing.

For the next two days, anger at God darkened my thoughts. It didn't seem loving for him to allow me to hope about the sleep study and not to give me any idea about where or whether I should go to find a diagnosis. I feared that I'd never know what was wrong and end up bedridden. Walking through God's beautiful autumn creation and gazing at it from the fourth floor of the library reassured me of his perfection and power, but I wasn't sure about his love. If he didn't love me, I was heading for disaster in this life and in eternity. If a perfectly wise and powerful god wouldn't make a good plan for me, how could I make one with my limited intelligence and strength? That would be harder than assembling a puzzle while its picture was still being painted. I didn't share what I was wondering about with anyone because this situation seemed between just God and me. But as hours passed, I sank into despair at the thought of handling life with a chronic illness.

I sat on my bed Saturday evening, gazing at the greasy-haired, frowning girl in the mirrored sliding doors of the closet because I couldn't do anything productive. Then it hit me, or God hit me with it: if I couldn't trust the almighty and omniscient God, I couldn't trust anyone or anything.

So I needed to trust him. I'd have nothing at all if I didn't have him. My burden was too much for my family and me to bear alone. It was clear that I'd fallen into an inaccurate, negative thought pattern I'd learned to recognize through counseling. Just because I thought that I'd never have a diagnosis and that no treatment option would succeed didn't make either true.

After a few more days and many prayers, I decided to pursue a diagnosis of CFS or something similar. Mom had researched Mayo Clinic, while I had researched Cleveland Clinic, which Beth knew was excellent from personal experience, possibly better than Mayo. The Mayo Clinic had no CFS specialist, but I identified a Cleveland Clinic doctor who had an interest in fatiguing illnesses. Besides, Cleveland was closer to home. To start the referral process, I needed another appointment with Dr. Three. I scheduled it for my birthday, in October, because I'd be home that weekend.

I went home for one weekend each month, tops, because of the draining, time-consuming drive. It wasn't even a hard drive. I set my cruise control for almost the entire ride through farmland and didn't have to maneuver through four-way stops until close to home. Even if the drive had been easier, I wouldn't have gone more often because I needed all the spare time I could get to rest, do enough homework to pass my classes, and talk with friends. Every time I didn't feel up to calling one of the twins to chat, it bothered me because my friends were strong supporters. I didn't want to lose their support or friendship.

I was in danger of losing not only friends but also my stimulant that semester because of a nationwide shortage of it. I'd heard about the shortage, and then one day the campus pharmacy didn't have enough of the medicine to fill my latest prescription. My home pharmacy had none of it. I called every pharmacy in Mount Pleasant, where my college was. That amounted to about six pharmacies because Mount Pleasant is bigger than Flushing but isn't a big city. The staff and approximately 26,000 students at the time made up roughly half the population, and Soaring Eagle Casino and Resort was its only other major attraction to outsiders. Pharmacies that had the stimulant wanted to reserve it for their current customers. I called other pharmacies in my hometown and found one that could supply me. I mailed my scrip home to Mom so that she could have it filled. Unfortunately, Dr. Three had forgotten to write his provider ID number on the scrip, a requirement for stimulant scrips, so the pharmacy refused to fill it. That required Mom to drive half an hour to Dr. Three's office to have him add his ID number to the scrip.

By then, I had so few of my pills that I was taking half doses. I didn't need this extra stress. Although you're not supposed to send medicine in the mail, Mom sent the stimulant once she got it. She couldn't deliver the medicine because of her jobs, and I couldn't spare the time and energy a drive home midweek would've taken. I can understand that rules concerning how to write prescriptions and concerning not mailing medicine are in place to prevent drug abuse. But they also can prevent sick patients from getting the medicine they need.

The next month, the same scenario happened, with two exceptions. First, Dr. Three remembered to write his ID number on the scrip, and second, I never received the package Mom sent containing the medicine. This wasn't the only time I failed to receive mail at my apartment, and I never had the time or energy to investigate, another illustration of how likely people with disabilities are to tolerate injustice. I wasn't sure whether it was even worth the trouble to get the stimulant because it didn't help as much as it had before. Taking just half a dose of it hadn't affected my functioning much, and some days I forgot to take my second dose in the afternoon.

Fortunately, my October appointment wasn't far off, so I got a new scrip then. During that appointment, I planned to get a referral to Mayo or Cleveland Clinic. After I mentioned this intention to him, we reviewed everything I'd undergone at the U of M.

Dr. Three then said something that changed my life: "It's time for us to start calling this and treating this like chronic fatigue syndrome. That's what you seem to have."

It was a wonderful birthday present. I don't recall ever saying "chronic fatigue syndrome" in his presence, so for him to confirm my deep-down suspicion was surprising. No, it wasn't a certain diagnosis, something he could point to on a lab report. No, it wasn't the diagnosis I'd wanted, because I'd wanted something easily treatable. But it was a *name*. The warm flame of relief brightened my mood more than I'd thought it would. On the way home, I thought, *How will I learn to live with chronic fatigue syndrome?* Then I answered my own question with a smile: *Duh, I'm already learning. I've reduced my activities to prioritize my health over school and work, allowed my parents to help me, and stopped being a go-getter.*

Dad, ever the pessimist, was puzzled by my smile when I told him the news. He reminded me gloomily that CFS has no cure.

Yes, that was true, but I explained that Dr. Three had a treatment to try: four to six months of antibiotics. The theory behind this treatment is the body thinks it's fighting an infection or something, causing the symptoms, so taking antibiotics should make the body think the infection is gone and quit acting weirdly. I didn't get my hopes up about this treatment. I'd learned to quit getting my hopes up about anything because of the heartbreak that followed when such hopes were crushed. I emailed Gramma, my friends, and my Writing Center supervisors that evening to share my diagnosis and antibiotic regimen.

For my birthday, my parents gave me a special white noise machine that played sixteen sounds, depending on the effect I wanted: relaxation, sleep, renewal, or tinnitus relief, not that I had to worry about that, which I was thankful for. I experimented with it for the next few weeks. It seemed to help me fall asleep faster, but the sounds labeled *renew* didn't energize me.

I thought, *Well, if this is my new life, it's not so bad*, as I got cheerful and supportive replies to the emails I'd sent on my birthday. Beth replied in person on Monday when I was about to enter the library Writing Center location.

"So, you got a diagnosis!" Beth said with a grin.

"Yes I did!" I answered with a bigger grin. I told her about the treatment I was trying.

"It's just a treatment, not a cure?" she asked.

"Right, no cure. There is no cure for chronic fatigue syndrome. Very, very few people, I think 5 percent, fully recover, based on what I've read. But I'll take *any* improvement!"

I kept researching CFS along with treatment and coping methods. I grew to prefer the combined name ME/CFS. *ME* stands for myalgic encephalomyelitis, whose root words break down to mean muscle pain with inflammation of the spinal cord and brain. Say it with me: my-ALL-jick en-SEEPH-uh-lo-MY-eh-light-is. ME sounds more legitimate than chronic fatigue syndrome. *Fatigue* is too gentle a word for what I experience, and probably everyone experiences fatigue lasting more than a few weeks at some point. People also equate the symptom with drowsiness, and I'm *not* drowsy or sleepy. I feel more like my brain is firing on half its cylinders with fumes in the gas tank. One online ME/CFS discussion board said antibiotics and antivirals were outdated treatments that rarely worked. I frowned but kept taking my antibiotic, even though it caused nausea if I forgot to take it with a snack, caused sunburns in December, and wasn't helping my ME/CFS. I thought maybe it would help my acne, which had improved somewhat but was still severe enough to be embarrassing. A medicine-related article I found on the discussion board interested me more. It explained that ME/CFS patients often experience the opposite of what certain drugs, including antidepressants, are meant to accomplish. We don't metabolize drugs the way healthier people do. Finally, I had assurance that the first antidepressant I had taken had caused my depression.

My dreams began reflecting my feeling of entrapment in my body. One night, I dreamed that to get out of dreamland, I had to relive my three previous dreams but change something in each. For one of those three dreams, the change was to drink every liquid in sight. Even when I woke up, drenched in sweat, I was convinced that I had to fall asleep to finish the bizarre task. When morning came, I had to take a shower because of all the sweating. I also had multiple nightmares about evil doctors preparing to operate on me without anesthesia.

I couldn't help but think of the doctor nightmares as I waited to see Dr. Three one day in December. First two and then four of my fingertips had developed little hard bumps weeks ago. Ointment wasn't helping. Dr. Three said he'd never seen anything like these bumps. He prescribed an antifungal and then an antiviral when that didn't work. The latter seemed to help. The bumps yellowed, flattened, and flaked off. I hoped this was a onetime occurrence.

Starting the spring semester was difficult emotionally. Life was much easier when I lived at home, where Mom did the cooking, laundry, and cleaning. It was as hard for Mom and Dad to let me return to school as it was for me to go. Dad's coping mechanism was napping, and Mom's was giving me a cooler full of frozen meals and then cleaning until I called to say I'd made it to Mount Pleasant. Mom told me more than once she wished that she could keep me home to take care of me, but I knew if I quit school, I'd return only if I received a cure for ME/CFS. I knew how unlikely that was. If I wanted to have anything resembling a career, I needed my degree. I wanted to make financial contributions to my family in exchange for living at home after graduation and to be a worthwhile investment of my scholarship providers' gifts.

As I attended my first spring classes, barely able to listen to the routine overviews of the syllabi, the shadow was obviously heavier. I suspected I was sicker because I hadn't rested enough during a weekend trip to Chicago with my parents and brother after Christmas. One morning we had walked an indirect route from the Bean to the Hancock building without stopping. My suggestion of getting a cab had been ignored, so I'd thought it was pointless to ask to stop and sit. It had been foolish to hope that my condition wouldn't worsen once I had a diagnosis. I estimated that I was functioning at 35 percent of the level I had when I'd been well. The antibiotic wasn't helping, but Dr. Three had said to give it more time when I had seen him during Christmas vacation.

One day during the first week of the semester, Dad called me as I was walking to the shuttle bus to my apartment complex. During our conversation, Dad asked, "How many hours are you doing this semester?"

"Nine," I answered.

"No, I mean credit hours," he said.

"It's the same. Nine."

"That's all?" He sounded surprised.

"That's all I can handle," I replied firmly, trying not to take his question as criticism of my work ethic. I doubted that he understood just how miserable I felt every day. After we hung up, I prayed, "God, please help Dad understand how I feel, and forgive me for my negative attitude toward him."

As the weeks passed, even with the reductions in activity I made, busy days often drove me to tears. I gave up on exercising more than thirty minutes in one day because it drained me and because I needed every minute of rest I could get. By *exercising*, I don't mean going all out in a gym. I mean walking slowly from class to the bus stop and maybe doing some squats in my bedroom. Exerting myself physically even slightly more than usual caused muscle or joint pain the next day. I stopped making pancakes, once a treat, because of how much it would wear me out, and I bought microwave dinners after resisting doing so ever since moving out of the dorms. I also depended on the frozen leftovers Mom sent back to school with me every time I came home. Although I didn't like unloading those coolers of food after the taxing drive to my apartment, I appreciated not having to cook many meals. My roommates were always gone or busy (one working or shut up in her room with her TV blasting, the other working or partying) when I arrived, so they couldn't or wouldn't help unload.

Even my personal hygiene was starting to suffer. I couldn't do all my laundry in one day because of my low energy and because the dryer was so wimpy that it took at least two cycles for clothes to dry. I kept my laundry bag in the closet to keep it away from one roommate's highly lovable but nosy dog, so any clothes hanging there probably smelled like dirty laundry. Old underwear stank because of my discharge. On a few evenings, I lacked the stamina to take a shower. I couldn't make that chore less draining by sitting or kneeling in the stall, though I tried both, because the textured floor was painfully rough. I didn't feel up to shopping for a shower seat or want to inconvenience the roommate I shared the bathroom with.

The cognitive exhaustion frustrated me more than the physical exhaustion. I was becoming more easily distracted and having more trouble remembering what I'd been doing after any disruption. I nearly stuck the broom into a bucket of water and more than once opened Microsoft Word to send an email. Sometimes, I felt like I was sleepwalking because I wasn't taking much in as I moved. Formerly I'd been observant, watching for people and situations that could inspire scenes in stories I wanted to write. On bad days, I felt almost brain-dead as I absently hummed while trying to read for class or said the wrong word, such as *mass* when I meant *mess*. More than once I recalled a scene in *Flowers for Algernon* where the temporarily highly intelligent protagonist realizes he's losing his intelligence and pictures himself returning to being a custodian with a vacant grin as a little tune plays. Some patients call the cognitive troubles *brain fog*, but I felt like I had a *brain barricade*. Or maybe a brain brick wall, seeing as that sleep lab technician had thought there was one at the back of my nose. Like an old computer, my brain took forever to boot up in the morning, had a small amount of memory, and tended to lock up if I did two actions at once. I tried hard not to worry or feel guilty if I skipped a class or a chapter of homework, but the habit of being a good student was the most difficult to break. Actually, *crack* is a better word because I'd somehow achieved all As the previous semester, unless I chalk that up to grade inflation.

I kept feeling pain in my fingers as I took notes one day. The bumps on my fingers had returned two weeks after their disappearance, even though I was still on the antiviral. Clearly, Dr. Three didn't know what they were, so I wanted to see a dermatologist. The dermatologist in Mount Pleasant didn't take our insurance. Because Mount Pleasant is in a county full of farms, the next closest dermatologist was farther away than I wanted to drive. I didn't trust Flint-area dermatologists. I'd grown to believe that because Flint is an unpleasant place to live, good doctors don't live or work here. Mom stepped in and scheduled an appointment to see a dermatologist at the U of M during my spring break.

Sometime that winter, I tried light therapy. I hadn't read anywhere that this would help ME/CFS, but I thought I might get a mood boost from it because it can treat seasonal affective disorder, a form of depression occurring only during a certain season, usually winter. Central Michigan University's (CMU) clinic had a special lamp that I could sit in front of for a half hour per week for only a few dollars. I wasn't surprised when I felt no different, but I wasn't upset, because the cost was so low.

In early February, I came down with a cold. Having even a cold on top of ME/CFS is worse than miserable. Viruses deplete my energy even more and take twice as long as normal to go away. By three o'clock on February 9, 2012, I'd already given up on doing any homework, cooking, cleaning, or anything that involved physical or mental effort. The *only* reason I went to my classes was out of guilt for the money my parents were withdrawing from their retirement savings to pay for them. Mom and Dad were paying about a third of my educational expenses.

In my English seminar class, we were discussing how students and faculty spend their time. Some students admitted that they didn't put their full effort into their classes because of their extracurricular activities and jobs. I also didn't put my full effort into school, but my reason was medical. The thought saddened me. I thought about my future, how money would always be a problem because I wouldn't be able to work full-time. Plus, I'd have medical expenses to pay, no matter which of President Obama's health care reforms were upheld as constitutional.

At the end of class, I had a little time before the next bus to my apartment complex came. I sat on a bench around the corner from the classroom, set my backpack on my lap, and put my head down on my arms on top of my backpack. I hadn't had a full fifteen minutes of rest yet that day, and my custom is to take one such rest period each morning and afternoon. I decided to pray for five to ten minutes and then catch the bus.

I prayed, *Please give me release, no,* relief. *I meant* relief. *Please give me relief. I'm ready to give up. I don't know how this is all going to turn out, but it's going to turn out for my good. Help me.* My nose began running, and I sniffed. *Please.*

"Are you all right?" a man asked.

I hadn't heard him coming. I lifted my head and saw that it was my professor, a thin man in his thirties with brown hair. His office wasn't this way, so I was surprised to see him.

"I thought it was you, I wasn't sure. It's easy to just walk by," he said quickly.

"Oh, I'm just really, really tired and wanted to rest," I answered, straightening my back some and trying to smile.

"Are you not getting enough sleep?" There was his charming British accent.

"Well . . ." I glanced to my left and right and saw no one else around. That gave me the courage to tell him the whole truth. "I'll tell you something about myself. I have chronic fatigue syndrome."

"Ah, that's debilitating." So he believed it was a real illness.

I remembered his comment on a reading response in which I mentioned Dr. One calling me crazy: "I know what you mean." I'd appreciated that comment but hadn't thanked him for it.

"It's amazing I'm still in school." My voice wobbled. I couldn't look attractive with my too-long bangs in my eyes and my loose ponytail, and crying wouldn't help. I hadn't had the energy to get a haircut.

"I know." I could tell he meant it. "My brother had it. Ten years. Then it went away." I hunched again slightly at the thought of spending ten years like this, and he put out his hand in a *stop* gesture. "Not saying that you'll have it that long. How long has it been going on?"

"Two and a half." It sounded far too long to me.

"Two and a half? Are you on any medicines?"

"Yeah, but they don't work." I thought, *That antibiotic is never going to help.*

"That's hard. And they're just now considering it a real illness . . ."

"Yeah, even my own doctor, well, I wrote about it in that response."

"I remember."

Wow, I thought.

He mentioned the couches upstairs, saying they would be more comfortable if I wanted to nap, and I explained that I had to catch the bus soon. He asked about my diet and whether I'd found any sort of support group.

More important, more than once, he said, "If there's anything I can do for you, let me know."

Just stopping was the best thing he could have done, showing me he cared. He walked on, saying he was headed to the library to get some coffee at the coffee shop inside. Astounded and relieved, I stared at the door through which he went. *Thank you, Jesus!* At once, I remembered what I'd prayed for and realized that I'd experienced an instant yes response to prayer. Then I cried.

Nearly a month later, spring break came. Unlike many of my classmates, I didn't travel out of state. Instead, Mom and I drove to the U of M for my appointment with the dermatologist. He was as handsome as you'd expect someone of his specialty to be, with a perfect complexion and thick brown hair, appearing maybe five years older than I. He examined and squeezed my fingers and called the mysterious bumps chilblains.

"Chilblains? What are they?" I asked.

"They're bumps caused by poor circulation, which makes sense, seeing as you have Raynaud's," he explained. "*Pernio* is another name for them. A lot of times, they're seen not necessarily with Raynaud's, but with autoimmune diseases, like lupus. Were you tested for autoimmune diseases before you were diagnosed with chronic fatigue syndrome?"

"Uh-huh," I answered, but I started to feel uneasy at his concerned look.

"How long ago were those tests?" he asked, letting go of my hand to take notes.

About ten seconds later, my memory finally supplied the answer: "Almost a year ago."

"Hmm. I'm just wondering because, when you're so young, sometimes things like lupus can take years to show up on blood tests. It takes time for the antibodies to reach a level that the tests can detect."

What? Why the heck was a dermatologist, rather than all the other internists and specialists I'd seen, informing me of this? The dermatologist recommended that I see a U of M rheumatologist he knew of who specialized in lupus. He offered to make the referral for me. I agreed that I should see this doctor to double-check that I didn't have an autoimmune disease.

I also had the dermatologist examine my stubborn acne. He was somewhat surprised that my antibiotic hadn't helped it, and he prescribed two creams to apply twice daily. Those helped slightly but would've worked better if I'd had the energy to apply them in both the morning and the evening every day. Because I tended to mix tasks, I also had to be careful that I put the creams on my skin, not my toothbrush.

With the dermatologist's revelation came the possibility that my diagnosis was incorrect. I'd rejoiced over knowing what was wrong. Now I'd been thrown back to the darkness of square one, or at least square two. The mistakes and oversight of medical professionals I'd dealt with frustrated me. Every day on which I didn't get a phone call with the date of my appointment with the lupus specialist added to my impatience. I needed treatment *now*. I felt like my life was on hold, and I was sick of listening to the crummy music.

I sent an email about my new doubt to Gramma, my friends, my academic adviser, and my Writing Center supervisors. When the director of the Writing Center emailed back first, sending hugs and telling me not to give up, my eyes filled with tears. This shows how exaggerated my emotional responses can be when I'm this weary. Before getting sick, I never cried at sad parts in movies, in church, or when feeling grateful. Now I do.

Once I finally had the appointment, I felt suspended in deep space. I didn't want to research lupus in more detail because it would be a waste of time and energy if that wasn't what I had. I didn't want to research ME/CFS clinics or treatments because it would be a waste of time and energy if *that* wasn't what I had. I couldn't afford to waste time that I needed for classes and homework. I wished that I could've taken six instead of nine credits, but then I wouldn't have been able to graduate in December. At the same time, it was frustrating to feel unable to improve my health until that appointment on April 27. It was also stressful, no matter how much yoga or deep breathing, two activities I'd turned to as coping methods, I did to try calming myself. Yoga helped only by making me notice where I tensed muscles and wasted energy and by being a form of exercise I could attempt on bad days. I also began overchewing my food, a digestion tip I'd read online, which had no effect.

Gramma's timing for sending an uplifting card was perfect. Inside it, she wrote, "We get so impatient waiting for an answer from God, but His timetable isn't like ours. Don't ever give up on Him." It's cruelly ironic that an adjective that doesn't describe me, *patient*, is also a noun that describes a person seeking medical care. I have never been and never will be a *patient* patient.

I came close to being an emergency room patient on the last day of my spring break. I returned to the apartment Saturday evening to have a day of recovery from the drive and organizing before classes resumed. I felt extra tapped out and sad as I unpacked what I had to unpack that day, such as the newest batch of leftovers Mom had spoiled me with. The thought *I don't want to be here* wouldn't stop repeating, even when I tried distracting myself by watching funny videos online. I was alone because my roommates wouldn't return until the next evening. When I cried later, I went to bed early.

The next morning, the sadness and exhaustion remained, accompanied by a feeling of sparks shooting through my brain periodically when I moved. I wasn't sure I should drive, but I decided that going to church would lift my spirits. I wound up unable to concentrate during the service because even blinking sometimes caused brain sparks. By the time I got back to the apartment, I felt chilly and shaky and barely had the energy to pour a big bowl of cereal for my lunch. I wasn't hungry, but I hoped that food would help. It didn't relieve the shakiness, making me wonder whether I had a fever. I didn't have a thermometer. I would've gone to bed, but it was probably still damp from the severe night sweats I'd had that night. I needed to wash my bedding and finish unpacking yet couldn't force myself to move. I started crying, thinking, *I want Mom.*

I didn't get up from the table until I had to use the bathroom. I took my comforter and blanket off my bed but couldn't do anything more, so I sat on the bed and considered calling Mom. I didn't like calling on bad days because I made her worry. But I'd never had a day this bad, so bad I couldn't determine what was wrong or what to do. After some time, I gave up and called home. Dad answered, and I told him how I felt. It didn't sink in right away.

"You'll be all right. Just put the laundry in the washing machine and take a nap," Dad suggested.

I managed to sigh instead of cry. "I don't feel up to it. I feel really sick." There was a pause.

"You want to talk to Mom?"

"Yes, please." I told her the same thing I'd told Dad, and it seemed to sink in during the pause that followed.

"Do you want me to come up?" she asked.

I momentarily hated myself, but it seemed like the only option. "I think I do. I'm sorry."

Mom sighed. "Okay. Give me time to pack. I'll probably spend the night, so I'll need to call and have someone else make the bank deposit for me tomorrow morning."

I couldn't blame her for sounding disappointed. I forced myself to put my bowl and spoon from lunch into the dishwasher and then plopped onto the blue couch. Even though I couldn't fall asleep—the insomnia had been flaring up for a few days—I stayed there until Mom knocked on the door a little before three o'clock. She took one look at me after hugging me and told me to sit down, so I went back on the couch. Her hand on my forehead detected no fever. She called Dr. Three, who was on call, fortunately. He recommended taking me to an urgent care center to make sure my heart and lungs were working properly, but without my chart in front of him, he couldn't remember my medical history.

The physician's assistant at the urgent care center found normal vitals, a normal urinalysis, and a high blood glucose reading (more than 200). She had blood sugar and complete blood count tests ordered for the next morning and said I should rest today and see my endocrinologist if I didn't improve in a day.

After Mom and I went to Qdoba for a quick dinner, we returned to my apartment, and she did the laundry and even the vacuuming that I'd also intended to do that weekend. The brain sparks stopped before we went to bed. The next morning, I felt relieved of the previous days' worst symptoms as soon as I took off my sleep mask. I sat up and smiled at Mom, who was putting her earrings in.

"Well, you're smiling. That's improvement," she said a tad grumpily, but after what I'd put her through, I couldn't blame her.

"Much better," I answered, getting out of bed without feeling like I was going to faint or have a seizure. We went to the hospital to have the bloodwork done and then went out for breakfast. While we ate, we brainstormed what had brought this on: a missed dose of a medicine, the insomnia, a mild case of an acute illness, or simply a really bad day. I'd been so careful about taking all my medicines because I was desperate for them to work, but maybe my poor memory had won this round. I'd gone from home to school without becoming so ill before, so I doubted that emotions had brought on all the symptoms. Mom asked me whether I could handle being at school.

"I don't want another bad phone call tomorrow," she went on. "I can't skip work tomorrow. If this is too much for you, I'll take you home with me today."

She meant that if I went home, I wouldn't return, but it took only a few seconds to make my decision. "I'll be okay now. I'm so sorry I made you do this, and I really appreciate it."

For months, we lived in fear of another day like this. In retrospect, I think that terrible day was the result of some combination of the causes Mom and I had listed over breakfast. We'll never know because I've never had another day that bad. My blood tests came back normal, so the high blood sugar had been temporary. I did experience brain sparks one day months later when I took my antidepressant a few hours late. I learned that surviving a chronic illness is probably impossible without support from family or friends and gave up on being financially and geographically independent from my family.

CHAPTER FIVE:
The Shadow Grows Heavier
☙

After weeks of impatience and frustration, I saw the second rheumatologist in May, the one the dermatologist had recommended. I had nine vials of blood drawn for testing. At least I think it was nine—I felt woozy during the eighth one and lost count. All the tests came back normal. False alarm. It was a relief to learn my condition wasn't an autoimmune disease, except for the nagging questions of "Now what?" and "Does this mean I have ME/CFS?" I couldn't imagine Cleveland Clinic or Mayo Clinic being able to do much more for me than the University of Michigan (U of M) had.

Months earlier, I'd searched online for clinics that specialized in treating ME/CFS, so once the semester was over, I returned to the notes I'd compiled from the search results. By the end of the summer, I wanted to handle my ME/CFS better and feel improvement. As I researched the clinics further, I learned most used only one treatment protocol, which was often named after the doctor in charge. The single-treatment approach made me think, *Suppose so-and-so's treatment doesn't work for me?* I wanted a clinic that would try multiple methods. Besides, the costs associated with these clinics were going to be high. The clinics were out of state, out of the Midwest, even. I didn't want to invest time, energy, and money into a trip to one of them, only to return home with no improvement or answers. I refused to subject my family, or myself, to that emotional blow. But not trying a specialty clinic seemed like giving up. I was too young to give up, so when I got an article about a multifaceted ME/CFS treatment approach from a radiologist at church, I was inspired to try it.

The article was written by ME/CFS specialist Dr. Jacob Teitelbaum. He explains the illness as a blown fuse in the brain, the fuse being the hypothalamus, which regulates body temperature, hormones, hunger and thirst, sleep, blood flow, and other variables that maintain balance in the body. One element of Teitelbaum's protocol was vitamin B_{12}. I knew vitamin B_{12} shots by themselves had helped other patients. Maybe the shots or other elements of the protocol would work for me, and I wouldn't have to go to a specialty clinic. I drew boxes around paragraphs I wanted Dr. Three to read and scheduled another appointment with him for June 1, 2012, to share the article.

Three days before the appointment, something happened that made me think I'd see Dr. Three for another reason. I was riding my bike to Kroger, which was almost directly across the street from my apartment complex, and had the idea to make a sharp turn and then go up a steep hill. This is more evidence that I wasn't as smart as I had once been. I didn't have enough momentum and crashed sideways, tweaking my handlebars permanently and throwing much of my weight onto the wrist that had been hurting off and on for over a year. By the time I returned to my apartment, that wrist was already swollen and throbbing, so I figured I'd sprained it. One of my roommates helped me get a bag of ice on it as I scolded myself.

The next day, the swelling was already down enough to where I could wear my brace. My wrist didn't hurt as much, which relieved me because I had to work at the Writing Center. That would require typing as I worked with students in online degree programs. At the end of my shift, I took the brace off and rotated my right hand four times clockwise and then counterclockwise to stretch my wrist. To my amazement, I felt no pain, though that same motion had caused pain nearly every time for the past year. I rode the elevator with Beth, who was also working at the Writing Center that summer, her final semester. I told her what had happened.

She grinned and said, "Maybe you should fall off your bike more often—"

"Yeah, see if that cures the rest of my problems," I said, knowing where her joke was heading. After that day, my wrist didn't hurt. I thought my fall had popped something that was slightly dislocated back into place permanently.

I considered sharing Beth's joke with Dr. Three as I waited for him on the day of my appointment. After we greeted each other, I explained what I truly wanted to talk to him about.

"My chronic fatigue syndrome has gotten worse over the course of this year, and the antibiotic isn't doing anything. I'd like to try something else. I read this article, and I thought you should, too." I handed him a copy of the article.

"Chronic fatigue syndrome," he read aloud from the title. Then, he looked back at me and asked, "Could you summarize it for me?"

"Well, it's about the approach one specialist uses to treat it. He thinks a problem with the hypothalamus is the main cause. He focuses on improving sleep, natural steroids, and vitamins and minerals, like vitamin B_{12}."

"I don't want to give you steroids. Too many side effects."

"Okay," I said, a little surprised that he wasn't looking at the article.

"You know, I've mentioned you to some of my other patients. I didn't say anything bad, of course, just that you're having all these problems, and nothing seems to be helping. I've been working on a program for my patients. It officially starts tomorrow, but I've been swamped with people coming in wanting to start it today. I can give you an information packet about it if you want. It's based on the raw foods diet. Are you familiar with that?"

"No."

"It's heavy on fruits and vegetables. You don't cook them at temperatures above 116 degrees because otherwise you decrease the nutritional value of the food and degrade the enzymes. Now, starting the diet is a little rough because you're basically detoxing yourself. You might feel more tired. If you start this program, there will be required lab work beforehand and required visits to check on you while you're detoxing. But I've read tons of research about this, and they're seeing great results, not like all the other fad diets I've seen where you lose weight and then just pack it back on because your metabolism slows down. That's because your body thinks it's starving, and you end up doing a yo-yo. With raw foods, people are losing lots of weight, and it's treating high blood pressure, diabetes, autoimmune disorders, and so on. People with diabetes are able to go off insulin. There's no drug, nothing I can do to make people not need insulin anymore. That's incredible.

"I can get you an introduction packet and a video about raw foods today. Then if you decide you want to do it, call and make the appointments, and we'll get you a packet with a bunch of the research on this and instructions for doing the program. You've got to follow the instructions. We want to make sure you get through the detox part okay."

"I don't know about this. I don't think I could handle the detox," I said, getting confused.

"But it could really help you," he insisted. "In all my years of practicing medicine, I've never seen a diet with results like this. And we'll help you do this with our program. I've spent months developing it with the help of my fantastic business manager."

"But you don't know if this can help chronic fatigue syndrome."

"Studies show the raw foods diet helps autoimmune disorders. Chronic fatigue syndrome falls into that kind of category."

"So, you're saying chronic fatigue syndrome is an autoimmune disorder?" As far as I knew, ME/CFS didn't have a classification. It's a multisystem illness.

"Well, what causes it?"

"No one knows for sure. There are theories, but—"

"No. Chronic fatigue . . ." He stopped when he saw my bewildered expression.

"I'm sorry. I, I don't understand what you're saying. Say it again," I said.

"Well, here's what I'll do." He cleared his throat. "I'll get you the introduction packet and the video, and you can decide if you want to do it."

"Okay. What about the antibiotic? Do I need to keep taking it?"

"No, you can stop," he replied, scribbling something on my chart. "Let me get you that stuff, and I'll be right back." He left the room, leaving the article I'd brought him behind, and I looked at Mom, who looked confused as well.

The fact that he'd barely looked at the article and then been pushy, which he'd never been before, upset me. It was like he hadn't listened to anything I said and didn't have a clue how to treat my condition. For the first time, a doctor rather than an acquaintance had suggested that I try an unusual treatment that wasn't specifically for ME/CFS. As we drove home, we agreed that Dr. Three had been rude and that this diet didn't sound like a good idea.

"It might be good for weight loss, but you don't need to lose weight," Mom pointed out.

"Plus, the last time I changed my diet and went on that gluten-free deal, I got way worse, not better," I added, wishing that I'd thought to say that to Dr. Three.

"I don't know why he tried to push that on you," Mom stated for about the third time.

"Maybe he was so excited about starting that program that he couldn't resist running it by us. I don't know."

"Do you think we should even bother watching that video?"

"I don't know. Maybe we could. I just don't know what we should do now. If this is how he reacted to an article by a CFS specialist, I wonder if he'd even be willing to refer us to a specialty clinic, if we decide to go to one."

"I wish I could pack you up and take you to Mayo," Mom said, bobbing her head for emphasis every few words. It wasn't the first time she'd expressed that desire, along with the desire to get me a high-tech full-body scan that would pinpoint what was wrong with me.

"But I don't think they can help me. They don't have anyone who specializes in CFS," I reminded her.

"I wonder if he's even sure you have CFS."

"What else could I have? They've ruled out everything else."

We didn't watch the video. That night, I wrote in my journal after a tear slipped out of one eye, "Doctors shouldn't be allowed to make people so miserable." I wouldn't have been as upset if Dr. Three had just admitted that he didn't know how to help me or just listened to my concerns. Doctors can't treat a patient with invisible problems if they don't use their ears to listen to what he or she says more than what the heart and lungs sound like.

I was ready to give up on doctors and treat myself, based on supplements I'd read about that had helped other patients. Never had I been so sick of and *from* doctors. All those months on the antibiotic had been a waste. I had no clue what to do. I knew I didn't want to see Dr. Three again, but that was about it. Sure, I had multiple options, including finding a new doctor and going to a specialty clinic, but I didn't know whether it would be worthwhile to try any of them.

I searched for patient reviews of the ME/CFS clinics on third-party websites. It was eye-opening to find as many negative reviews as positive reviews. A couple of patients revealed how much one clinic had charged for initial evaluation and treatment, which was information that hadn't been clear on a few of the clinics' websites. The clinics didn't take insurance. I'm grateful to those patients who weren't afraid to share this information and their frank opinions. A visit to a specialty clinic would have a price tag in the—gulp—thousands of dollars. Not just two or three thousand, either. I couldn't make my parents pay that when money was already tight. I couldn't risk spending all that money and time and then feeling no better.

I could tolerate living the way I'd lived the past three years and pray that I didn't end up bedridden. Through a free online self-study course Bruce Campbell and Dr. Charles Lapp created for people with ME/CFS and fibromyalgia, a disease I consider a cousin of ME/CFS, I was learning strategies for managing my illness better. For instance, I started brushing my teeth and applying sunscreen while sitting down and stopped trying to multitask. I wrote down my personal rules for managing my condition, such as "Plan your day as if it's going to be a bad day," which made them feel more authoritative. Before, I had known that multitasking wasn't good for me but felt that I had to try it on busy days. I attempted to care less about anything upsetting, such as a dirty bathroom, because even emotional responses sucked up energy. After reading about the value of having routines, it dawned on me that I thought more clearly in mornings because of my clear routine. Later in the day, deciding what to do next could paralyze my brain for ten minutes. I'd been indecisive even when I'd been healthy.

Though the course's strategies didn't improve my physical well-being, I was a little less frustrated because I was doing *something* to make life easier. I finally understood that my illness was one I couldn't fight in the sense of trying to keep living the way I had when I'd been healthy. The course brought out that the more I fought like this, the worse the illness would get. To some extent, patients have to take ME/CFS lying down. We're not professional athletes who have to play through the pain. I needed to pace myself by determining how much energy I had on a typical day and exerting myself only that much every day. Before, I'd made myself work so hard on weekdays that on weekends I could barely function. It was like I was overdrawing a bank account all week long and then having to pay overdraft fees on weekends. If I knew I had something extra to do on a certain day, I started doing less the days before and after that rougher day to help balance my energy budget.

Something else I tried that the course didn't mention was caffeine pills. Mom thought they might help me get through bad days. After taking them three times, I gave up on them. They didn't help during the day, and then I couldn't fall asleep until well after midnight. I took the pill in the morning, but it obviously didn't get out of my system until late at night. That didn't make sense to Mom. But the light bulb went on when I read something that month about

ME/CFS patients having sluggish livers and other digestive dysfunction.

Alongside learning to manage my illness better, I was considering my doctor situation. I wanted to switch primary care physicians after what had happened with Dr. Three, but I couldn't find any clinic whose receptionist expressed confidence in the physician's ability or willingness to work with an ME/CFS patient. This added to my frustrations. I was never truly angry or sad about having ME/CFS or envious of healthy people. But I experienced frustration daily: frustration with the lack of a cure, frustration with the health care community's lack of knowledge about the condition, frustration with doctors who wouldn't listen, and frustration with my limitations. I didn't know any way to make that emotion vanish besides finding a good treatment for my ME/CFS.

On June 17, I did one more online search for ME/CFS specialists in Michigan, Indiana, or Ohio whom patients benefitted significantly from. I didn't want to travel beyond those states. I found one right in Michigan with positive patient reviews on more than one website. She was both a regular doctor and a naturopath, so it seemed like she'd balance conventional and complementary medicine in her practice. As I understood the term, a qualified naturopath has as much training as a medical doctor and focuses on using natural approaches to prevent and treat illness. After looking over the clinic's website, I called the office and left a message, saying I was considering seeing the specialist and had questions.

Two days later, while I was praying for guidance, especially as to whether I should try this doctor, the clinic's receptionist and nurse returned my call. She answered my questions about the doctor's experience, amount of time spent with patients, and treatment approach—smart questions to ask when considering seeing a specialist. The specialist regularly attended conferences and read journal articles concerning ME/CFS. She spent an hour during the first appointment and half an hour during follow-up appointments and prescribed both medicines and supplements. She did not use a one-size-fits-all approach with her name attached to it. One of my other questions, asked in light of what had happened with Dr. Nutrition and after seeing supplements mentioned on the clinic's website, was whether the specialist sold the supplements she recommended. It turned out she sold them only if they were hard to get otherwise. The answers were satisfactory enough for me to schedule an appointment.

After I hung up, I debated whether to go through with the appointment. That night I wrote in my journal, "I feel sure about the appointment." I reread the sentence. *Wait, I meant to write* unsure. *Was that a mistake, or is that what I really feel?* I wrote faster, "I wrote 'sure,' and I got the phone call during prayer . . . but I thought the sleep study was a sign from God." *And look how wrong I was.* "I think this doctor will be the last one I try."

It was hard not to worry about what would happen during the appointment. In fact, I had more than one nightmare involving doctors during the two-and-a-half-week wait. I'll call her Dr. Special. During the drive to her clinic, which took almost three hours, I had a thought that put a positive spin on my fear that she wouldn't be good: *at least if the experience is a letdown, I didn't have to wait long for it to be over.*

Her small clinic looked more like a home. The waiting area had a striped couch, which I sank into because just riding in a car that far had worn me out, and an electric fireplace between two cushioned chairs. The nurse apologized for making me stand up just as I'd settled on the couch and took me to an examining room that had a curtained window with a view of the woods in front of the building.

Dr. Special had mostly gray hair that fell to her shoulders and wore glasses low on her nose, a long skirt, and casual flats. She looked at a list I'd made of all the treatments I'd tried. When she saw D-Ribose on there, she asked whether I'd taken the powder itself or the full D-Ribose protocol. Dr. Nutrition had prescribed the D-Ribose, the powder supplement meant to boost energy.

"I didn't know there was a full protocol," I replied.

"Well, for best results, four other supplements have to be taken with D-Ribose: carnitine, CoQ10, magnesium, and malic acid," she explained.

That was a strike against Dr. Nutrition. I started to write down the other supplements, knowing I'd forget them otherwise and fearing Dr. Special wouldn't wait for me to finish writing because most of the doctors I'd seen had been in a rush.

But she said, "Don't worry about trying to write them all down. I'll write down for you what to take, the dose, and the frequency." Wow, she realized that I had cognitive difficulties and that she needed to spend more time with me than the average physician did.

Also, the way she nodded at or guessed what symptom I was describing when I mixed up my words, instead of giving me a blank or puzzled expression, showed her understanding of ME/CFS. She also understood when I described the effort I'd put into researching ME/CFS after finding my doctors' knowledge of it was minimal.

When she looked down my throat, she announced, "Yep, you've got them. Crimson crescents. Did you ever come across them in your research?" I shook my head, and she explained that they're reddish, crescent-shaped markings seen near the tonsils that indicate ME/CFS. More than 80 percent of patients have them. Her discovery boosted my confidence in her and in the accuracy of my diagnosis.

She told me to start the D-Ribose protocol; eat more protein; drink water with electrolytes daily because of my excessive sweating, which made me think, *Duh, why didn't I think of that? Darn brain fog*; and start vitamin B_{12} shots. She recommended that I get the serum from an out-of-state pharmacy she was familiar with, explaining that its price was lowest, and have a nurse at the campus clinic show me how to do the injections on my thigh. That way I wouldn't have to exert the extra energy to go get them twice a week.

Dr. Special even expressed a desire to make my life easier by offering me a handicapped parking permit, which I declined. I'd read at least one account of someone with an invisible disability being challenged or having his or her car scratched after rightfully parking in a handicapped space. I didn't want to be next, and I'd never collapsed while walking across a parking lot. Finally, Dr. Special gave me a flyer for a ME/CFS and fibromyalgia support group. Although it met in Grand Rapids, too far for me to drive from school or home, I was sure that I could ask to get on its mailing list and check out any resources it had on its website.

During the drive home, I reflected on how the appointment had been like bright, beautiful stars coming out at night. But I reminded myself that every doctor I'd seen had seemed kind and able to help during the first appointment, wanting to make a good impression. Doctors seemed to show their true colors during the second and third appointments. When next month's appointment with Dr. Special came, I'd feel more confident in judging whether she was worth seeing long term. The next day, Mom verified some of what Dr. Special had said by finding the crescents in my throat and an article about them by Robert B. Marchesani online. Crimson crescents were discovered back in 1992, so it seemed like by now, doctors besides ME/CFS specialists should've known about them.

When I had requested copies of my medical records from the U of M and Dr. Nutrition for Dr. Special, I had requested extra copies for my reference. I wanted to know what the other doctors' impressions had been and whether any lab results had been abnormal or close to it. They had arrived so close to my appointment date that I hadn't had time to look at them beforehand. A note on the U of M labs caught my eye: they'd been done at the Mayo Clinic. I was glad I hadn't gone there, then, because its doctors probably would've done the same work the U of M doctors had. Going to a state-of-the-art hospital or clinic doesn't guarantee better care because good technology can't compensate for a doctor who lacks compassion, comprehensive knowledge, or curiosity, in that order.

This became clearer when I looked over the lab reports from Dr. Nutrition. He had told me that I was deficient in pregnenolone, vitamin B_{12}, and potassium and that my vitamin D and white blood cell counts were low. However, unless he'd meant to say that the levels were lower than what he'd *like* to see, he'd told the truth about the white blood cell count *only*. My potassium and pregnenolone levels were on the low end of normal. My vitamin B_{12} and vitamin D levels were well within the normal range. I can tolerate a doctor's occasional mistake, as long as it doesn't endanger a patient's life, because we're all human. But I cannot tolerate a doctor lying to me, especially when his reason for it seemed to be to justify selling more products to me. Let me repeat a lesson I mentioned earlier: examining copies of medical records is a good way to see if doctors are missing or covering up anything.

I acted on other information Dr. Special had given me by emailing the leader of the ME/CFS support group, and along with adding me to its mailing list, she emailed me a folder with informational files. One of the files described diagnostic criteria for ME/CFS that I hadn't seen before. Bruce M. Carruthers et al. published these criteria, called the International Consensus Criteria, in 2011. The criteria required patients to have postexertional malaise and categorized the other symptoms doctors could use to make the diagnosis, clarifying that the illness has to affect multiple body systems to be ME/CFS. The categories were neurological (at least three symptoms required for a diagnosis); immunological, gastrointestinal, and genitourinary (at least three symptoms required); and energy production and transport (symptoms in this category include sweating and dizziness upon standing, and one symptom must be present). Combined, the symptoms had to cause a reduction of one's activities by 50 percent. These diagnostic criteria are more accurate than the criteria in the Mayo Clinic's CFS article because someone with depression or a neurological disorder could be misdiagnosed as having ME/CFS easily under the old criteria. I went online to see if the Mayo Clinic had updated its criteria and found that it had, but they weren't the same as the International Consensus Criteria. These differing sets of criteria must be confusing for those few physicians out there who want to learn about ME/CFS.

I had done this reading about ME/CFS while waiting for the supplies to do the vitamin B_{12} injections. The campus pharmacy didn't carry needles and syringes and told me to try a medical supply store. I found one in Mount Pleasant, only to have its staff tell me a pharmacy should supply me instead. Irritated, I tried the local Kroger pharmacy and learned that it had the syringes but not the needles in stock. I'd already ordered the serum, and it arrived from out of state before Kroger got the needles. Once I had the supplies, I called the campus clinic to arrange to have a nurse show me how to inject myself.

"We could, but we'd need to have a statement from your doctor that authorized us to do that," the receptionist said.

I thought that was ridiculous. I was just asking a nurse to show me how to do a routine procedure. He or she wouldn't even have to touch me.

"Well, suppose I decide not to do the injections myself, then. Are you allowed to just go ahead and do the injection for me, if I bring in the serum, syringe, and needle?" I asked.

"We would still need a statement from your doctor authorizing that," the receptionist answered.

"Okaaay." I tried not to convey too much annoyance. "May I have my doctor fax that to you, or do you need it in some other form?" I thought, *Is Dr. Special going to have to hand deliver the statement or some fool thing?*

"It can be faxed. Let me give you our fax number."

I copied down the fax number and said goodbye. It was Wednesday, so Dr. Special's office would be closed. Even so, I left a message to explain that I needed a statement, still struggling to keep annoyance out of my voice. I'd been ready to get my first shot today, darn it. If this treatment was going to help, I wanted it *now*. Getting shots two mornings each week wouldn't bother me. From the summer before second grade until the first summer I was in Dr. Three's care, I'd received steroid shots every few weeks to relieve my seasonal ragweed allergy.

Still impatient, I called the campus clinic again the following afternoon to see if Dr. Special's statement had arrived. It hadn't. I decided to look for instructional videos on YouTube. Heck with the extra effort needed to go to the clinic. I found a few videos, and in one of them, a nurse practitioner demonstrated the process on herself and clearly explained what part of the thigh to target. Part of me thought I was foolish to rely on YouTube for medical information, but the rest of me wanted to start this treatment.

The next morning, July 18, I set up my supplies on my bedside table to avoid the exertion required to carry them to the bathroom. I slid the chair from my desk over to the table. Once I filled the syringe, it took a couple of minutes to work up the nerve to continue. The needle, 1.5 inches long, looked as long as a knife blade. I kept telling myself, *You can do this. Just do it!* I inhaled through my nose. As I started to exhale, I stuck the needle into my right thigh. Ow! I pressed the plunger with my thumb. Ow, ow, ow! This hurt more than any other shot I'd received. I paused and looked at the bottom of the syringe but couldn't see any blood there, so I kept going. It would have been hard to differentiate blood from the red wine–like B_{12} serum, anyway. I was alone, so I let myself cry, "Ow! Get it out of me!"

Finally, all the serum was gone. I pulled the syringe out and felt squeamish. "That hurt!" I exclaimed as I dropped it inside an empty water bottle on my bedside table. That's where I planned to put my used syringes until I figured out Mount Pleasant's medical-waste disposal rules. My leg wasn't bleeding, but I had a strange sensation of impending sickness. I knew what that feeling meant and was glad I was just one step away from my bed, where I plopped myself down to keep from passing out, trying to concentrate on my hot pink polka-dot comforter. My whole thigh ached. Apparently I'd hit a nerve. I kept telling myself I was being a baby. *I want to be stronger than this.*

After about ten minutes, I felt well enough to get up to throw away the syringe and needle wrappers. I could hardly walk, and that remained true for the rest of the day. I sure as heck wanted the injection to cause improvement, after the trouble and pain I was going through to administer it. Thankfully, that was the only time I hit a nerve. After feeling sore the next few times I injected into my right thigh, I decided to do the shots only on my left thigh and have Mom give them to me in the hip when I was at home. She knew exactly how to do that from seeing nurses give me allergy shots there. I learned another lesson to share with patients: *don't use YouTube or the Internet to learn how to do medical procedures.* Maybe I would've hit the nerve that day even if I'd had in-person instruction, and when I finally had a nurse show me in person where to inject myself, it appeared I shouldn't have hit a nerve. Even so, I'll never take the chance of hurting myself badly for the sake of convenience again.

By the sixth injection, I'd lost hope that this treatment was helping. Even so, I justified injecting myself every three days by thinking, *Maybe this will keep me from getting worse.* I estimated that I was functioning at 30 percent of my pre-illness level. I could handle worsening of the physical symptoms, but if the cognitive symptoms worsened much more, I'd probably lose my ability to work part-time as an editor once I graduated in five months. I'd long given up on working full-time. My reading comprehension was even worse than before. Some evenings, my concentration was so poor that I couldn't get anything out of reading the newspaper, and I felt brain-dead.

While telling God how I felt like a prisoner in my own body, a thought struck me: we who have problems with our bodies will probably marvel at our perfected bodies in heaven even more than those without such problems. This life and this body are only temporary. Even though I couldn't see how being ill would work out for my good, I trusted it would. As I was writing in my journal one evening, this encouragement struck me: I can't give up on God; he won't give up on me.

Another encouragement was slight relief from my night sweats. Mom's boss with fibromyalgia had heard of a brand of sleepwear made out of rayon, Cool Nights by Soma, which supposedly helps keep the body cool and dry despite sweating. Mom and I found an outlet store that carried the brand and bought some pajamas for me. The rayon felt cool and light, even to the touch, and reduced the number of times I woke up drenched.

A third piece of encouragement came from a second helpful appointment with Dr. Special as my final semester of college was about to start. I still didn't trust her fully, but she was the best doctor I'd consulted so far. She suggested using oxygen when I did mentally challenging tasks, such as homework. The idea was that if I got more oxygen to my brain, it would function better. I'd never thought I'd rent an oxygen tank at age twenty-two. Even so, I reminded myself that I was blessed in that respect. The oxygen allowed me to read one more page or write one more paragraph in one sitting. It wasn't enough to make up for how much my cognitive problems had worsened over the summer, but I was happy to have it. The oxygen made my nose cold enough to run, which opened my eyes to the negative experiences of people who have to use it regularly.

My last source of encouragement was my gut. My digestive problems were apparently gone, thanks to the D-Ribose protocol and to avoiding mushrooms and pain medicine for the past month. I'd noticed that I didn't seem to digest mushrooms and had episodes of loose stool within a day of taking an over-the-counter pain medicine for muscle or joint pain or headaches. I celebrated, and tested my digestive system, by eating a piece of chocolate cheesecake when Mom took me out to the nicest restaurant in Mount Pleasant during a weekend visit in September. I concluded after reviewing my illness timeline that when I'd been seeing Dr. Nutrition, D-Ribose, not avoiding dairy, had helped my digestive symptoms in the weeks before I'd stopped eating gluten.

Even with those few small gains, I decided never to bake or cook anything that required more than five ingredients or steps. Cooking and then doing dishes was already too much. This probably sounds strange, but I *wanted* to clean, to have the energy to cook and clean. Many evenings, I gave up on homework and cleaning and sat in bed with my laptop or some leisure reading. One night after I turned my lamp off, I found I lacked the energy to pull my comforter over me. Although I was taking only two classes that semester, searching for someone to sublease my apartment to and for a part-time job took much time and energy.

I wanted time for more fun activities—not parties because I'm not a party person, but maybe sporting events, creative works readings, and concerts, especially if Maria, one of my twin friends, would play her French horn. She would graduate after student teaching in the spring. Only about once per semester did I manage to spend a couple of hours just chatting with friends at a coffee shop. Maria had recently visited to give me a birthday present. I'd wanted to ask her to clean my room or make a meal for me. But I couldn't work up the nerve to do it, knowing she was busy, too. Would she have stopped being my friend if I had? No, but I perceived a greater chance of losing friends than of losing family by sharing my struggles with them. The college years are supposedly the best of one's life, and I didn't welcome the thought that those years were nearly over. I wondered whether after graduation I'd gain even the slightest pleasure from remembering college or remember only how grueling it was. I prayed that getting my degree while sick would be the hardest thing I'd ever do in my life.

That challenge encompassed several smaller challenges, such as becoming comfortable with the idea that I had a disability. I'd learned the government's definition of *disability* semesters ago in a management class, but I hadn't thought until now to approach CMU's Student Disability Services to see if I qualified for accommodations to ease my studies. I decided not to bother trying because I was so close to graduating. I was now used to thinking of myself as someone with a disability but not assertive enough to educate people I encountered who made insensitive remarks about people like me. For instance, one afternoon in November, I was sitting in a bus shelter on campus, waiting for a bus that should've been there fifteen minutes ago. Two women were in the shelter, griping about the bus. I knew their faces but not their names because we lived in apartment complexes on the same road.

"I guess the bus skipped us," one said glumly.

"Maybe it broke down," I suggested. "That happened to me once. It broke down at Wal-Mart, and it took them half an hour to get another bus to us. They just skipped the rest of our bus's route."

"Half an hour?" the glum one replied. "I would've walked home from Wal-Mart, yeah, rather than wait *half an hour*." She made my choice to wait sound ridiculous. From there to my apartment probably would've been a ten-minute walk with just one road to cross, after all.

"But I'm disabled," I chirped just as the other woman started to say something. "I have a disability," I corrected myself, remembering a booklet I'd read that explained the use of person-first language to describe people with disabilities. "I couldn't go that far." The glum one looked at my legs, searching for leg braces, I guess.

"I'm just lazy," the woman I'd interrupted said. "That's my disability—a mental disability, laziness." They both giggled.

I smiled and nodded slightly, choosing not to let that response offend me, though I disagreed that laziness constituted a disability. *Oh, honey, you have a lot to learn about disabilities*, I thought.

Then, I remembered another time a month or so earlier when I could've gotten offended after hearing something insensitive at church. I was talking with a man I knew but hadn't conversed with much before. Somehow I wound up saying I had a health problem.

"What do you have?" he asked.

I hesitated, accustomed to telling this only to people I knew well, but answered, "Chronic fatigue syndrome."

He laughed and said, "I have that, too." Maybe he noticed I was grimacing and not smiling, because he changed the subject. But I'm still not sure whether he thought I was joking. He moved away from the Flint area, so I never had another chance to bring up my health with him.

I had heard another insensitive, ignorant remark during the summer, this time from a doctor. I'd caught a bug that caused simultaneous vomiting and diarrhea. My inability to keep water down prompted worries about dehydration, so at about two in the morning I went to the emergency department by myself via ambulance, where I told everyone caring for me that I had CFS.

The emergency department doctor's response to that information was dismissive: "Oh, so you're wanting to sleep all the time?" Too whipped to tell him just how serious an illness CFS is, I said yes. This illustrates why ME/CFS is a better name for my condition. *Fatigue* is far too wimpy, and the power of the words we use affects not only how people characterize us but also how much funding a government gives to research a disease.

Maybe I missed good chances to educate the doctor, the man at church, or the women at the bus shelter. I've often wondered whether I should've told them, "My illness, and any disability, is nothing to laugh at. Shame on you. You're making what's already a difficult life for me worse." Saying that would've used up more energy, though. Maybe it wouldn't have made any difference, and maybe I would've caused them to think people with disabilities are mean and touchy, which isn't true.

Because I find being assertive is more important when speaking about disabilities with doctors than with acquaintances, I will say this now to doctors: if you don't know much about a medical condition, ask the patient how it affects him or her or how it should affect the care you give. Dr. Special does this when she asks which daily activities are most challenging for me and how long I can do a given activity. Don't make any illness sound trivial. I know it's hard for people to help someone who doesn't appear to need help. But doctors, of all people, need to think before they say anything potentially offensive to someone with a medical condition.

I wanted help when in mid-November, I had one of my bad days. I attended a Writing Center staff meeting despite the desire to skip it as I had the previous meeting, and I had to stay afterward to mention two important things to the director. I needed to let her know that I'd applied to two online tutoring companies because she was one of my references. I don't remember what the second thing was. When I stood up, I felt unsteady but made my way to her with my left hand hovering over seat backs in case I needed to grab one for support.

She looked at me, saying, "You look like you need a hug," and gave me a big hug. Apparently, I looked almost as bad as I felt. Normally only Mom could tell when I was having a bad day by either looking at me or hearing my voice.

That afternoon, I decided to suspend job hunting until after graduation because I was too overwhelmed. I tried to convince myself that I wouldn't miss any job opportunities because few companies would hire someone new this close to the end of the year.

I also hadn't found anyone to sublease my apartment to, so I was worrying about that. Even if I didn't find someone, I'd move back home as soon as my classes were done. I wouldn't participate in the graduation ceremony because of the cost and energy involved. My parents didn't mind missing a college graduation because they'd gone to Dwight's graduation in Kentucky at the end of the spring semester. I awaited going home to stay as eagerly as I imagine many elderly Christians await going to heaven.

The Saturday after Thanksgiving, I went out to breakfast at a local diner with my parents. As we were eating, Mom and I made eye contact.

"What's wrong with your eyes?" she hissed.

I wasn't aware of anything wrong with my eyes. I could see fine.

Mom looked at Dad, who was sitting next to me in the booth, then back at me. "Your pupils are huge," she said softly.

"Really? That's weird," I replied.

"His eyes are normal, so it's not the light," Mom continued. "It's creepy. People are going to think you're on drugs or something."

Dad looked at my eyes. "Ooh, yeah, they are big," he commented.

"I don't know why they're like that," I said, feeling uncomfortable. A minute later, I remembered reading something during the summer that mentioned pupil dilation.

After we got home, I searched for the notebook where I'd written notes from the self-study course I'd taken that summer. There was nothing about pupil dilation there, but at the end of those notes were other notes I'd taken from a book called *Treating and Beating Fibromyalgia and Chronic Fatigue Syndrome* by Dr. Rodger H. Murphree. Aha! According to the book, a way to test for adrenal dysfunction is to face a mirror and shine a flashlight into one eye. After thirty seconds, if the pupil starts dilating, you should suspect adrenal deficiency. If I understood this correctly, a body with insufficient adrenaline, secreted by the adrenal glands, can't keep pupils constricted during long-term exposure to light. Adrenal dysfunction contributes to ME/CFS symptoms. (If you're going to try this test on yourself, please read about it in his book first in case I've misremembered the procedure.)

I'd also noted that long-term stimulant use could cause adrenal burnout. Stimulating poorly functioning adrenal glands is like beating an injured horse to make it work harder. The horse, like the adrenal glands, will work for a time but eventually collapse under the strain. It looked like, despite decreasing my stimulant dose in August after sharing that very fear with Dr. Special, I'd used the medicine for too long. My digestion and speed in falling asleep had improved after decreasing the dose, again showing my sensitivity to medicines. I shared the information about adrenal deficiency with Mom and Dad during dinner. I developed the habit of looking at my eyes in the mirror at least once a day, and I kept seeing huge pupils, especially in the morning. It was creepy, as Mom had said, like I was constantly making Bambi eyes, like the invisible shadow was becoming visible in my eyes. Even worse, I wasn't sure whether we could do anything about them. They were my body's way of screaming at me to stop because this semester was too much for me, but I wouldn't stop when I was three weeks away from finishing school. I kept praying for strength and praying that I wouldn't end up bedridden after pushing myself through the last weeks.

I also feared that the effects of pushing myself this hard were harming Mom emotionally. Sometime that weekend, I had something insignificant to ask her and went into her and Dad's bedroom. My body forced me to sit on the bed even as my brain reminded me how long it would take to make myself get back up. After I asked my question and got my answer, I was a little surprised when Mom sat down next to me.

"I didn't want you to leave home and go far from me, and now you won't leave home after graduating. I wanted to quit one of my jobs after you graduated, and now I won't be able to, if you can't work," she said. "If making you sick was God's way of keeping you home, I don't like it. That makes this all my fault. I've prayed and prayed about you, but he doesn't do anything." This wasn't the first time she'd said my illness was her fault, but it was the first time she'd explained why she felt that way.

"Mom, I'm not blaming this on you," I stated firmly.

"It is. It's my fault, and it's such a mean way for God to treat you."

"Everything works out for our good. There's got to be a better reason for God to let me get sick than to punish you."

"A perfect God wouldn't do this to you."

Mom had brought me up in the Lutheran faith, so to hear her doubt God's perfection was worrisome and shocking enough to keep my brain from generating a response—until I remembered doubting God after hearing the sleep study results. Then I knew what I could say that might help her.

"There was a time when I doubted that God loved me," I began. "I finally realized that if I can't trust God, I can't trust anything or anyone. I'd have nothing at all if I didn't have God. Life would be completely pointless and hopeless." What I mean by that is without Jesus, there's no chance of having a better life after death.

Mom sighed. "I suppose."

She took my bike and most of my clothes and books home after visiting me the first week of December. December is her busiest month because one of her jobs is church secretary, so I appreciated her help even more than I would've any other time of year. Even so, it seemed like there was an awful lot to pack and load alone. The intermittent wrist pain had returned, complicating the task to the point where I considered throwing my weight onto my right hand the way I had when I'd crashed my bike that summer to see if that relieved the pain again. I didn't try, imagining myself saying to the doctor at the hospital, "I broke it by falling on it to make the pain go away!" I left some kitchen items for my roommates to avoid making another trip to my car.

I turned in my last paper and took my last exam without caring what grades I got on them. I said goodbyes at the Writing Center staff party and at an Advent service at church. I returned my oxygen tanks to the medical supply store. The morning I left, I wrote a farewell note for my roommates and gave the dog a long hug. All I remember about my final drive from Mount Pleasant the next day was that it was snowing lightly and that I lay down shortly after arriving to an empty house. I doubt that I had the energy to feel any emotion stronger than relief.

The shadow shrouds my memory of my first month at home. Unpacking my car took about two weeks. Shortly after Christmas, I caught a cold that forced me to spend more time in bed. I left home once or twice a week, driving only when I needed more supplements. Mom was happy I was home, because she could care for me rather than worry about me. Dad needed more time to adjust to my return, though. He once said something to the effect of "I thought the idea was that you'd move out after graduating." I guess he still thought I was going to recover soon and live a normal life.

True, going back home to Mom and Dad is something few if any college graduates boast about, but I shouldn't have felt ashamed. I had no intention of hanging out and playing video games instead of looking for work. Another lesson I'll share with chronically ill patients is that *there's nothing wrong with asking for major help in the face of life-changing events.* Man, I wish that someone had told me that when I first fell ill. Again, there's nothing wrong with getting help from family and friends. It's a good way to show love and strengthen relationships, and being independent is an American value, not an American law. Determination helped, but I would not have graduated without the support of my family, my professors, Dr. Special, and my friends.

I received my diploma in the mail in January and reread three words of it while feeling proud: not *Bachelor of Arts*, but *Magna Cum Laude*, meaning "with high honors." My cumulative grade point average was 3.8. Those words, I suspect, are more of a testament to compassionate English department professors who inflated my grade after I explained that my illness kept me from putting my full effort into their classes than to my own ability. But I still felt thrilled to see those words on that piece of paper I'd worked so hard for. I was struggling to function, often spending an hour or two in bed in the afternoon and longer than that on the couch daily and sleeping between nine and ten hours at night. Mom worried when she came home from work and found me on my side on the couch, too worn out to stand up to greet her, so pale that, according to her, I looked ready to pass out. She told me later that she'd wanted to take me to the emergency room on some of those days to be sure my heart and lungs were working. I'll never forget the couch's brown pinstripe because I spent that much time staring at it rather than the pages of the books I tried to read. At night, when I was ready to go to bed, Mom often pulled my hands to help me get off the couch and onto my feet. I feared that this diminished functioning was a permanent effect of pushing myself too hard the last weeks of the semester.

While sitting in bed and on the couch, I read more about biological factors of ME/CFS when I could concentrate. I say "biological factors" instead of "causes" because it's uncertain what makes each organ system go awry and in what sequence. Organ systems are interrelated and affect each other. For example, much of the immune system lives in the intestines, so digestion can affect immunity and vice versa. ME/CFS impairs mainly the neurological, immune, and endocrine systems. The immune system reacts abnormally to a viral, bacterial, fungal, or environmental trigger and becomes less effective. Problems with the interworking among the brain's hypothalamus and pituitary gland and the adrenaline-secreting adrenal glands, called the HPA axis, damage the endocrine system and brain, causing symptoms that vary from person to person. Genetic abnormalities and depletion of the most powerful antioxidant, glutathione, hinder removal of toxins from the body and impede cellular energy generation in those tiny mitochondria that years before I'd considered a possible cause of my illness. These processes make up how I've come to understand ME/CFS based on my readings, and yes, I know it's oversimplified.

I also spent time learning about the government's treatment of ME/CFS. For instance, from 1995 to 1998, the Centers for Disease Control and Prevention diverted $12.9 million meant for ME/CFS research to unrelated projects, according to a report by the inspector general of the Department of Health and Human Services. Even now, the report

"Estimates of Funding for Various Research, Condition, and Disease Categories (RCDC)" showed that 2017 was the first year the National Institutes of Health spent more than $10 million on ME/CFS research. The Scleroderma Foundation states that about 300,000 Americans have scleroderma, and $17 million was awarded to research it in 2017. A much higher amount, $111 million, went toward multiple sclerosis research in 2017, and the National Multiple Sclerosis Society estimates that this disease affects about 2.3 million people worldwide. In contrast, I've read estimates of the number of ME/CFS patients that range from as few as 800,000 to as many as 4 million in the United States. (I couldn't find Beth's Friedreich's ataxia in this report, but maybe funding for research of it is combined with another disease category.)

Clearly, the government isn't considering the number of afflicted people when determining how much funding to give ME/CFS. Maybe it would argue that because ME/CFS doesn't claim lives, it shouldn't receive research funding. I say being bedridden because of a disease we know too little about is *existing*, not *living*. My case is moderate, but those with severe cases remain bedbound and sometimes unable to communicate. The government is also ignoring how ME/CFS hurts the economy by costing 18.7 to 24 billion dollars annually in lost earnings, according to 2008 research by Leonard Jason, Mary Benton, Lisa Valentine, Abra Johnson, and Susan Torres-Harding. As I read about all of this, it was hard not to be discouraged, especially when I didn't know how my own case of ME/CFS was going to progress.

Finally, I felt better able to think, read, and move during February 2013, which made my job search more manageable. I refused to let my search last the national average length then—forty-two weeks, if I remember a Central Michigan University Career Services presentation correctly—even if that meant becoming a work-from-home transcriptionist instead of a writing tutor or editor. Besides, I needed money because my checking account was down to about $100, even after selling all my textbooks that were worth anything and a few fragments of gold. I was still paying the rent for the apartment because I never found a subleaser for it, and Dad refused to pay. Yes, he had the right to do so; I was worried and upset about that at the time yet thankful that he wasn't charging me rent to live at home. The next month, I was hired as a work-from-home transcriptionist, but I kept looking for a position where I could make my degree worth the effort I'd exerted to earn it. The next month, a publishing services company hired me as a independent contractor copyeditor. I was happy to have work in my field and the convenience of a freelance position. The work wasn't steady, but that was fine.

Then God provided a position that made me overjoyed in August: writing tutor at Baker College of Flint, a local private college. Here's why I was overjoyed.

CHAPTER SIX:
Lightening the Shadow
☙

I have deliberately waited to say what, besides my faith, uplifted me and kept me from dropping out of college after falling ill. If I had dropped out of school, I would've lost this refuge: the Writing Center. The Writing Center was the one place where I felt witty, on the ball, and energetic and could feel relief from my exhaustion. Each day, I was excited to meet new writers.

On one such day, in the Writing Center location in the basement of the building where English classes were taught, I met a typical student. I'll call her Kathy. After introducing myself, I let her lead me past a couple of smiling coworkers and round tables, toward the vibrant mural of Earth painted on the back wall. The mural's border comprised squares, each painted by a writing consultant to represent some aspect of writing or of his or her personality.

"How is your day going?" I asked brightly as we sat.

"Okay, I guess. Kinda busy," Kathy answered. She wore a plain black shirt and a tan plaid scarf. While digging through her purple backpack, she asked, "How are you?"

"Oh, pretty good, now that I'm here." I grabbed a square of scrap paper and pencil from the little wire basket on our table. "Have you been to the Writing Center before?"

"A couple times," she replied with a shy little smile.

"Okay, great! So, what are we working on?" I leaned forward and looked Kathy in the eye.

She glanced down as she tugged a folder out of her backpack. She said the assignment was a "problem paper." I thought I knew which English 201 assignment she was referring to, but I probed for more details, twirling the pencil in my fingers while paying attention to her words and body language. I'd become much better at understanding and communicating with others in the years I'd worked in the Writing Center. She was concerned about the organization and grammar of her draft. As I started to explain our practice of reading writing aloud, she interrupted to say she wanted me to do the reading.

"Sure!" I answered. "Feel free to interrupt me at any time if you want to talk about something. I won't be offended. And I'll probably stop sometimes, too. Ready?" Kathy nodded and smiled again. I read, and the sound added another instrument to the soothing orchestra of calm voices (most of them female), of fans above us, and of tapping computer keys.

The third sentence of the assignment was a run-on, more specifically, a comma splice, I felt out of breath by the end of it and I sucked in the air when the long sentence was over with at last.

"Oh," Kathy said, examining the sentence. "That was long. I should break it up."

"Yeah, I think readers would appreciate that," I replied. "Where do you want to split it?"

Later on, she stopped me again to ask whether what I'd just read made sense.

"Not quite," I responded gently. "What do you mean here?" She explained the idea more clearly than the sentence did, while I swiftly wrote key phrases on the scrap paper. "That sounds better to me," I commented when she finished. "I think you can write it like that." With help from the phrases I'd jotted down, she wrote what she had said.

"There you go! Definitely clearer than the original, don't you think?" I asked. I spotted *effect*, which should've been *affect*. "Oh, I see one *little*"—I hunched over the table slightly—"thing you could change. See *effect* here?"

Kathy nodded, lifting her pencil over the word.

"That's the noun form. What's the verb form?" I asked.

"Oh. *Affect*. Whoopsie!" Kathy answered with a giggle. "I have trouble telling those apart."

"My trick for that is to think of *affect* as a verb, or an action word. This works as long as you're not talking about psychology," I explained, writing down *affect* and *action* on my scrap paper and then underlining the first letter of both.

"They both start with *a*," Kathy said, realizing what I was getting at.

When the session was over, Kathy told me how much this had helped her and how she felt better about the assignment now. She thanked me as she picked up her backpack.

"My pleasure," I answered, thinking the word *ecstasy* would be more accurate. I popped out of the chair and walked with her to the front desk, where I signed her out.

My work there and now at Baker College's writing center has provided more relief and hope for me than any doctor has—even Dr. Special, who still helps me manage my condition and suggests treatments to try. I wish that I could fill a prescription for and ingest 30 years of writing center work. Making better writers is my calling, yes, but more important, it helps my myalgic encephalomyelitis. At the beginning of this memoir, I wrote that having this illness is like body slamming a brick wall, being five decades older, and being unplugged in the dark. Well, making better writers cushions the impact of the brick wall that I feel like I body slammed. It lets me feel like I'm in my twenties instead of my seventies. It's an outlet for me to plug in to when I feel unplugged in the dark. The shadow has little weight on me in the writing center, unless I work for longer than six hours a day. I don't have a complete grasp of why this work helps me, but one reason is the therapeutic effect of forgetting my health problems and serving others. Patients with chronic illnesses need opportunities to forget that they're patients and have new experiences, whether that happens through listening to music, reading, sculpting, coaching, or some other activity.

As much as I enjoy that escape, I can't always forget that I have ME/CFS. Nor do I want to forget, because I'm spreading awareness of chronic illnesses and invisible disabilities, especially ME/CFS. Only with awareness will people have the understanding necessary to make patients' coming to terms with their health problems easier than it was for me. The first step toward supporting patients with invisible disabilities better is to talk more about these problems so that patients don't feel so isolated and afraid to seek help. Also, maybe with increased awareness, doctors will become interested in researching the causes and treatments of these complex conditions and in treating these patients whose bodies are complicated but who are grateful for medical guidance. There are at least 17 million ME/CFS patients worldwide, based on a calculation using conservative global population and ME/CFS prevalence figures from Niloofar Afari and Dedra Buchwald. Millions more suffer silently because they have yet to receive this diagnosis. They all need informed care and research from doctors, and they need understanding and support from the rest of you reading this. Maybe by researching ME/CFS, understanding of other fatiguing illnesses and of fatigue itself could increase, leading to better treatments.

I know not everyone who has had to rebuild a life after developing a chronic illness has a writing center or an equally brightening, lightening place or activity. Maybe my case is mild enough that the lightening effect is possible. Think about how much worse off the millions with severe cases are if this is how badly ME/CFS affected my life. Stories of chronic illnesses don't have endings involving cures or heartwarming reductions of limitations that fit into the myth that with willpower and hard work, anything is possible. Not everyone will find positive aspects of life with a chronic illness or have the energy to remember them on bad days. We can be grateful that we're free from a certain symptom, but that doesn't mean we'd pass on being disease free if we had the choice. So, how can other patients rebuild meaningful lives?

Two steps have been most helpful for me. First, as weak as it may sound, *accepting the limitations chronic illness imposes and your new life and identity* may help you feel more in control. Asking, "Why is this happening to me?" didn't move me forward or make me feel any better physically or psychologically. The key to this acceptance after grieving for my previous life was to shift focus to what I know and can do rather than what I don't know and can't do because of my health. I learned this after watching *Soul Surfer* but wasn't able to articulate it then. Second, after accepting your new life and learning to manage the illness, *find a way to contribute to society*—for example, Beth invites physical and occupational therapy students to her home to learn about life with and the needs of patients with Friedreich's ataxia. The contribution can take the form of somehow benefitting your caregivers—for example, I make greeting cards to send to my extended family, saving Mom a little time each month. Even contributions made from bed can add value to life and be another form of escape from illness and a chance to regain some control over life. But manage your illness first to avoid becoming a burden on supporters when you try to help them, like I burdened my parents. Being dependent on others is different from burdening them. My parents would probably claim I was dependent, not burdensome, but I know often the reverse was true.

Dodinsky said these steps differently in his book *In the Garden of Thoughts*: "Be there for others, but never leave yourself behind. When you own your imperfections and you embrace your life, you become a better person." I interpret "own your imperfections" as "Admit it when you need help, and congratulate yourself every day you, with even a smidgen of dignity, get through an illness-related experience that you'd thought you wouldn't be able to handle." Beth inspired that interpretation by sharing a seemingly simple story about her being handed a specialty cup with a straw rather than a regular mug of hot cocoa, which for her marked a progression of her illness that she handled with dignity.

I don't know whether I'll worsen, improve, or vacillate between worsening and improving. I don't know whether someone will find a cure. I don't even know what name my disease will have because the name proposed in early 2015 that I liked for being easy to pronounce, systemic exertion intolerance disease, hasn't caught on. I don't know and don't focus on these things.

But I *do* know more now than I did when I first fell ill. I know I'll keep educating people about my illness. I know I'll continue to shape writers and my own writing. I'm not just sitting here, waiting for God to say, "Let there be light" to make my lightened shadow vanish.

BIBLIOGRAPHY

Afari, Niloofar, and Dedra Buchwald. "Chronic Fatigue Syndrome: A Review." *The American Journal of Psychiatry* 160, no. 2 (February 2003): 221–36.

Brown, June Gibbs. "Audit of Costs Charged to the Chronic Fatigue Syndrome Program at the Centers for Disease Control and Prevention." May 10, 1999. Accessed March 23, 2015. http://oig.hhs.gov/oas/reports/region4/49804226.pdf

Carruthers, B. M., M. I. van de Sande, K. L. DeMeirleir, N. G. Klimas, G. Broderick, T. Mitchell, D. Staines et al. "Myalgic Encephalomyelitis: International Consensus Criteria (Review)." *Journal of Internal Medicine* no. 270 (2011): 327–38.

Chronic Fatigue Immunodeficiency Syndrome Association of America. "CFS Fact Sheet: Basic CFS Overview: Chronic Fatigue Syndrome." 2008. Accessed March 20, 2015. http://www.nova.edu/nim/forms/cfs-fact-sheet-english.pdf.

Dodinsky. *In the Garden of Thoughts*. Naperville, IL: Sourcebooks, 2012.

Groban, Josh. "You Are Loved (Don't Give Up)." Reprise/WEA, November 2006, compact disc.

Health Grades. "Multiple Symptom Search Combinations for Fatigue." Accessed December 2011.

http://www.rightdiagnosis.com/symptoms/fatigue/symptom-search.htm.

Jason, Leonard A., Mary C. Benton, Lisa Valentine, Abra Johnson, and Susan Torres-Harding. "The Economic Impact of ME/CFS: Individual and Societal Costs." *Dynamic Medicine* 7, no. 6 (April 2008): 6. doi:10.1186/1476-5918-7-6.

Marchesani, Robert B. "Crimson Crescents Facilitate CFS Diagnosis." *Infectious Disease News* 5, no. 11, 1992. Accessed July 31, 2012. http://www.immunesupport.com/news/93/sum007txt.htm.

Mayo Clinic. "Chronic Fatigue Syndrome." 2009. Accessed June 2, 2009. http://www.mayoclinic.com/health/chronic-fatigue-syndrome/DS00395 (site altered).

Murphree, Rodger H. *Treating and Beating Fibromyalgia and Chronic Fatigue Syndrome.* 4th ed. Birmingham, AL: Harrison and Hampton Publishing, 2008.

National Institutes of Health. "Estimates of Funding for Various Research, Condition, and Disease Categories (RCDC)." May 18, 2018. Accessed July 23, 2018. http://report.nih.gov/categorical_spending.aspx.

National Multiple Sclerosis Society. "MS Prevalence." Accessed July 23, 2018. http://www.nationalmssociety.org/About-the-Society/MS-Prevalence.

Robb, AnnaSophia, Dennis Quaid, and Helen Hunt. *Soul Surfer*. Directed by Sean McNamara. Culver City, CA: Columbia TriStar Home Entertainment, 2011. DVD.

Scleroderma Foundation. "What Is Scleroderma?" Accessed July 23, 2018. http://www.scleroderma.org/site/PageServer?pagename=patients_whatis.

Teitelbaum, Jacob. "Tired All the Time? A Doctor's Own Cure for Chronic Fatigue Syndrome." *Bottom Line Personal*, May 15, 2012, 8–11.

Wall, Dorothy. *Encounters with the Invisible: Unseen Illness, Controversy, and Chronic Fatigue Syndrome*. Dallas: Southern Methodist University Press, 2005.

Appendix A:
Seven Lessons for Living with a Chronic Illness

1. Examine medical records to see if there's an abnormal result the doctor missed or something he or she is trying to hide.
2. Compile illness timelines for yourself and for physicians.
3. Trust yourself more than you trust health care professionals.
4. Don't use YouTube or the Internet to learn how to do medical procedures.
5. There's nothing wrong with asking for major help in the face of life-changing events.
6. Accept the limitations chronic illness imposes and your new life and identity.
7. Find a way to contribute to society or your caregivers.

Write your own lessons or rules for living with your illness below.

Appendix B:
Resources for People Who Have ME/CFS or Fibromyalgia

Campbell, Bruce, and Charles Lapp. *Treating CFS/FM Self-Study*. Online course. Accessed March 16, 2016. http://www.cfidsselfhelp.org/online-courses/treating-cfs-fm-self-study.

MEAction. http://www.meaction.net/

MEPedia. http://me-pedia.org/wiki/Welcome_to_MEpedia

Murphree, Rodger H. *Treating and Beating Fibromyalgia and Chronic Fatigue Syndrome*. 5th ed. Birmingham, AL: Harrison and Hampton Publishing, 2013. (Disclosure: I copyedited this edition.)

Verrillo, Erica F. *Chronic Fatigue Syndrome: A Treatment Guide*. 2nd ed. Williamsburg, MA: Erica F. Verrillo, 2012.

ABOUT THE AUTHOR

Darla Nagel is a copyeditor and college writing tutor from Michigan. She blogs for chronically ill patients and their supporters at www.darlanagel.com.

www.ingramcontent.com/pod-product-compliance
Lightning Source LLC
Chambersburg PA
CBHW071927290426
44110CB00013B/1512